Table of Contents

Acknowledgements	3
Dedication	5
Birth Stories	7
Forewords	11
Introduction	14
Ffion's Story	29
Amy's Story	35
Lucy's Story	39
Anonymous	43
Seren's Story	51
Emma's Story	59
Eleri's Story	69
Natasha's Story	71
Kimberly's Story	75
Becky's Story	79
Charlotte's Story	87
Melissa's Story	93
Holly's Story	99
Siana's Story	105
Chelsea's Story	111
Jennifer's Story	115
Kate's Story	119
Kathryn's Story	123
Megan's Story	129
Kath's Story	135
Kath J's Story	141
Rosie's Story	147
Vicky's Story	155
Samantha's Story	163
Amanda's Story	167
Conclusion	179

1

Acknowledgements

A very sincere and heartfelt THANK YOU to all the Women & their families who very generously shared their birth experiences during this extremely strange and surreal time.

Equally, a very big thank you to the Head of Midwifery Julie Jenkins for kindly approving me to compile this collection of Birth Stories.

Can I extend my thanks to the Hywel Dda University Health Board for their consent to publish these Birth Stories.

Also, a very big Thank you to Emma Mills, Consultant Midwife, ABUHB for very patiently answering all my endless questions!

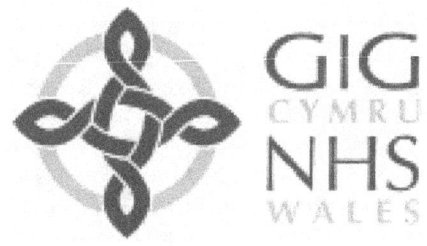

Dedication

Dedicated to all the women and their families who very kindly shared their very unique birth experiences during the Covid-19 pandemic

'Thank-you'

Also to all the Midwives, Doctors, Anaesthetist's, Theatre Team, Health Care Assistant's, Domestics, Paediatrician's and Special Care Staff who cared for them

Birth Stories

The following Birth Stories have been written by the women who gave birth to their babies in Wales during the covid-19 pandemic of 2020. The majority of the stories are based in the Hywel Dda University Health Board. Where any names and photographs have been included in the birth stories – it is with the prior consent of the women. The stories are raw, open, honest and moving accounts of their experiences.

I hope you enjoy reading them…

Birth Stories During the Covid-19 Pandemic

By Suzan Roberts

Forewords

Pregnant women and their families would have experienced a number of changes to a usual pregnancy over the COVID 19 pandemic period. COVID 19 has resulted in a considerable amount of the support being virtual, with the hospital and community advice changing constantly. It's challenging because it's new for all of us, but as a Maternity team we have figured out how to support and advocate for women and their families the way we normally would. The NHS and all its staff have been simply amazing at being so adaptive in ensuring we meet the woman's needs during these unprecedented times.

I am grateful for all the women and their families in giving their precious time to share their wonderful birth stories during COVID 19. These birth stories can be of benefit to almost anyone because it is something that unites us all as human beings: emotions. We have continued to focus our maternity services in at Hywel Dda University Health Board on a person- centred approach, promoting safe and high- quality care throughout this Pandemic period. To all the women and their families who have shared their wonderful humane stories thank you very much

Julie Jenkins
Head of Midwifery and Women's Services,
HDUHB

Covid 19 resulted in an unprecedented response within UK healthcare and for maternity services a passion to try and make, what is a life changing moment for women and their families in ordinary times, as positive as possible. Women and staff dealt with what was sometimes hourly changes in recommended practice and what personal protective equipment to wear with patience and sometimes humour.

Within Hywel Dda, along with services across the UK, we did our best to ensure that all choices of place of birth remained an option for women, and whilst the environments may have changed with transforming our alongside midwife led units into Covid areas the principles of midwife led care remained the same in our relocated areas. We are justly proud that at no point did we have to withdraw home births as an option, and in fact saw a marked increase as the weeks went by.

Some of us have learnt new technology skills and there are aspects of care that have been introduced during this time that may well stay, such as clinics run over video links where a physical check is not required and video link training for staff.

All staff went above and beyond to maintain choice of place of birth and to try and make every woman's experience as positive as possible, we are proud of every single one of them, from domestics, porters, administration staff, maternity support workers, midwives and doctors (across all disciplines).

What we saw was true team spirit, with everyone supporting each other as we all took turns to worry about not just the women and their families but also what the potential impact may be on ourselves and our own families. We are proud to offer this collection of birth stories as an insight into an unprecedented time in maternity care and what it's like to have a baby during a pandemic in West Wales.

Cate Langley, Consultant Midwife, HDUHB

Introduction

In the early months of 2020, we started hearing news of an epidemic that was taking place in Wuhan China. It was a respiratory illness that was compared to the SARS Virus. In the news it was reported that the illness was potentially fatal and spreading rapidly, prompting the Chinese authorities to put the entire region of Wuhan into lockdown.

By early February'2020 there were eight confirmed cases of covid-19 in the UK and subsequently the first confirmed case of coronavirus in Wales. China continued to report soaring cases.

Only a few weeks later, March saw the World Health Organisation declare a Global Pandemic of the Novel coronavirus (SARS-COV-2). By now, News reports from Italy also recorded a numerous number of cases with hospitals overrun beyond capacity, prompting the Italian authorities to declare a strict lockdown in certain regions.

As coronavirus cases also started to escalate in the UK, the British Government followed suit and by the end of March all schools were closed, GCSE's were cancelled, and National Lockdown started. Such unprecedented times saw the UK Government start a furlough salary scheme in a bid to keep people at home and minimise social contact, there was panic buying in the shops and queues to get into supermarkets. Pregnant women were included in the most 'at risk' category and advised to self-isolate creating fear and apprehension in all women expecting their babies. Fortunately, it later became apparent that pregnant women and their un-born babies are at no higher risk from the coronavirus than the general population.

Lockdown continued throughout May and on into June, the news was dominated with controversy about testing, with much debate on the reliability and efficiency of the tests.

Globally, by April there were over a million cases of coronavirus reported. In the UK alone the death rate was over 15,000 by the end of the April. Sadly, by the end of June, that was figure had increased to over 40,000.Thankfully, the rate of new cases started to slowly decline. As coronavirus numbers continued to decrease lockdown gradually started to ease throughout the UK during June and July.

As the contrary nature of the coronavirus became apparent during the pandemic, the news reported how some suffered serious symptoms resulting in critical care admission whereas other could test positive and have no symptoms at all. The seemingly random and indiscriminate presentation of the virus made it especially challenging, and the strict measures of lockdown and social distancing became all the more important.

In response to the global pandemic the NHS made a

huge effort throughout the UK to extend its capacity in order to meet the potential demand from sick patients. Medical and nursing staff were re-deployed from non-essential services back onto the wards, medical students were asked to start working on the wards, recently retired Health care professionals were asked to return to clinical practice, and field hospitals were set up in such venues as leisure centres and schools. Seventeen field hospitals were set up throughout Wales to cater for potential demand.

Changes in the Maternity Services across the Health Board due to Covid-19

In response to the Covid-19 Pandemic the Maternity Services in West Wales made numerous changes. Taking a multi-disciplinary approach across the Health Board, it adapted infrastructure and adjusted rotas across both the Midwifery and Obstetric workforce in order to ensure maximum safety for all. Both the rate and extent of the changes was certainly impressive, from Managers to Medical students, Anaesthetists to Admin staff and Paediatrics to Porters, we all worked together to make and maintain the necessary changes.

As a team, we took every possible precaution to keep the women, their families and each other safe, we endeavoured to support women's birth choices and keep things as 'normal' as possible – considering the circumstances and despite the PPE!

The Maternity unit was divided into two separate zones. The Red Zone was for any women with suspected or confirmed coronavirus and the all the other areas were considered Green zones. All women were screened for symptoms over the phone prior to admission and had their temperature checked on arrival. As the Midwife Led Unit was being used as the Red Zone, it was relocated to a different area so Midwives could continue to facilitate in giving women Midwife Led Care throughout labour, albeit the provision of waterbirths was unavailable at this time.

For the Community Midwives the screening process was done over the phone prior to any home visits, or Antenatal clinic appointments. As women endeavoured to stay away from the hospitals, the pandemic saw the Community Midwifery workload increase, as the rate of homebirths rose from 4% to over 12% during the first six weeks of lockdown.

As well as this, the Community Midwives also continued to support women giving birth in the Freestanding Midwifery-led Unit at Withybush General Hospital which maintained its normal function, although water births were not available during the pandemic.

To maximise safety and minimise the risk of transmission, we followed clear national guidance on wearing the personal protective clothing (PPE). In the Midwife Led Units, Labour ward and Home deliveries in the first stage of labour, gloves, a plastic apron, a fluid repellent mask were worn for basic care.

For the second stages of labour and delivery we had a long-sleeved gown as well as an apron, gloves, mask and a visor -it was certainly challenging! Especially when it was hot!

In response to the lockdown measures, and minimise the spread of the virus, and adhere to social distancing the Health Board had to take the difficult decision to limit all hospital visiting. The implications for the women and their families, meant having to forego the opportunity of having loved ones with them to share so many of the special moments and during labour they were limited to only having one birth partner. For pregnant women due to give birth during such testing times it was a particularly daunting prospect.

However regardless of all of this, they all dealt with the situation with patience and good humour, courage and strength which pays testimony to the many sacrifices they all made in order to adhere to the difficult restrictions imposed upon them through the coronavirus. Phone calls and video-calls were very much encouraged to try and maintain virtual contact with their friends and family.

Similarly, for the staff, we also turned to technology, video-calls for staff and training meetings replaced face-to-face meetings – which turned out to be a great success!!

Now lockdown is easing, it is a time for Maternity services to reflect, crunch the data and analyse the figures, admissions and attendances, outcomes and experiences. It is essential we listen to women's birth experiences in order to aid the shape and development of Maternity services of the future.

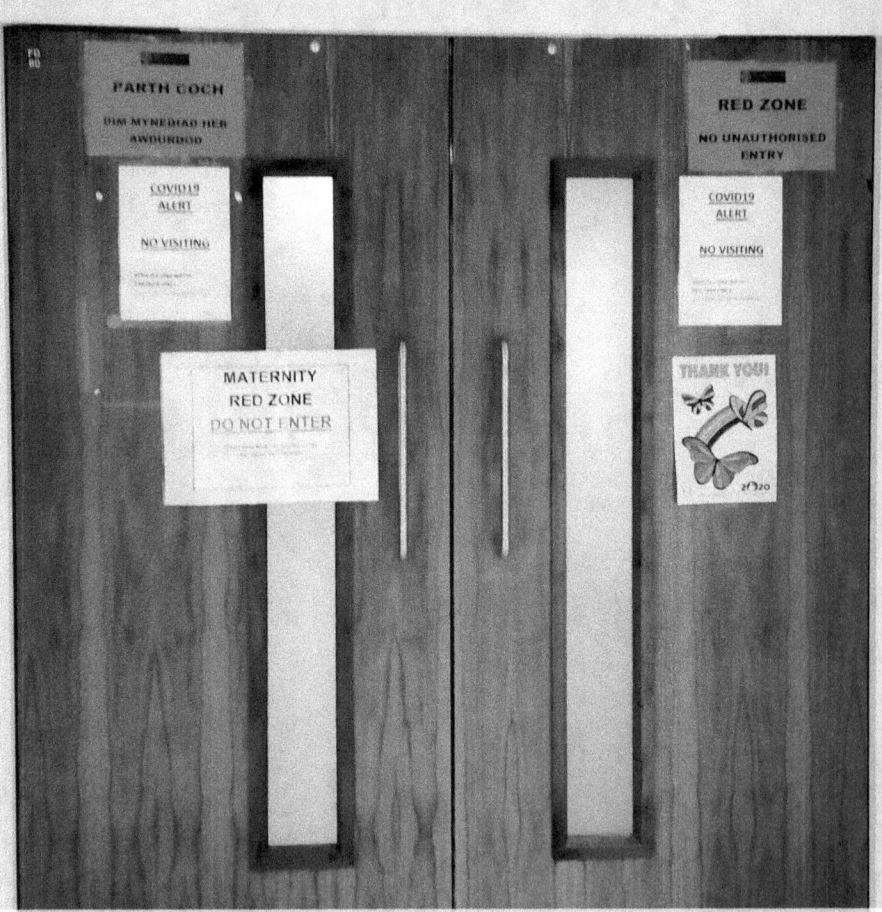

The Red Zone utilised in what was the Midwife Led Unit Carmarthen

Inside the Red Zone with a picture of appropriate PPE

DONNING AREA
(CLEAN ROOM)

COVID19 DONNING PPE (Theatre) CHECKLIST
TO BE CARRIED OUT IN THEATRE CLEAN ROOM

N.B Before donning any personal protective equipment, please make sure you have the correct theatre attire on – scrubs, disposable hat, hair completely covered, bare below the elbows. Empty pockets and perform hand hygiene. HAVE YOU HAD A DRINK AND COMFORT BREAK?

STANDARD PPE
(non sterile, non AGP)
1. Don apron
2. Don surgical face mask, making sure fit is snug
3. Don non-sterile gloves

FULL PPE
(non sterile, AGP)
1. Don surgical gown (t drops if possible)
2. Don FFP3 mask, check fit
3. Apply visor
4. Don sterile gloves

SCRUB STANDARD PPE
(sterile, non AGP)
1. Don surgical face mask, making sure fit is snug
2. Visor (or mask with visor)
3. Pick up sterile gown and your sterile gloves
4. Take in to scrub room
5. Carry out usual scrub routine

SCRUB FULL PPE
(sterile, AGP)
1. Don FFP3 mask, check fit
2. Visor, make sure strap is flat
3. Pick up sterile gown and your sterile gloves
4. Take in to scrub room
5. Carry out usual scrub routine

Before entering theatre –
- Ensure all PPE is comfortable. Do not adjust PPE while in theatre.
- Do not touch your face or any non-essential items.

Inside the Red Zone, more PPE instructions

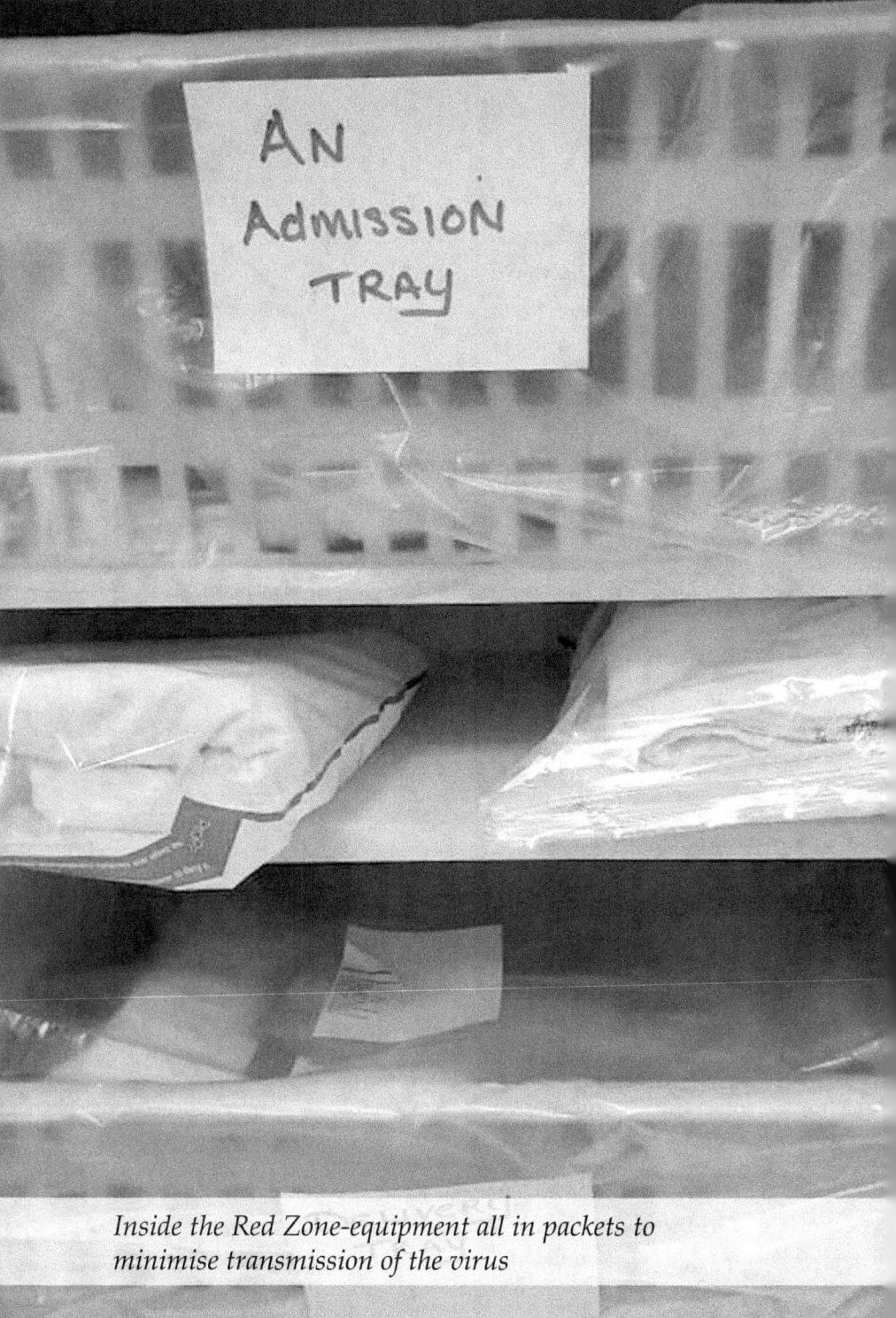

Inside the Red Zone-equipment all in packets to minimise transmission of the virus

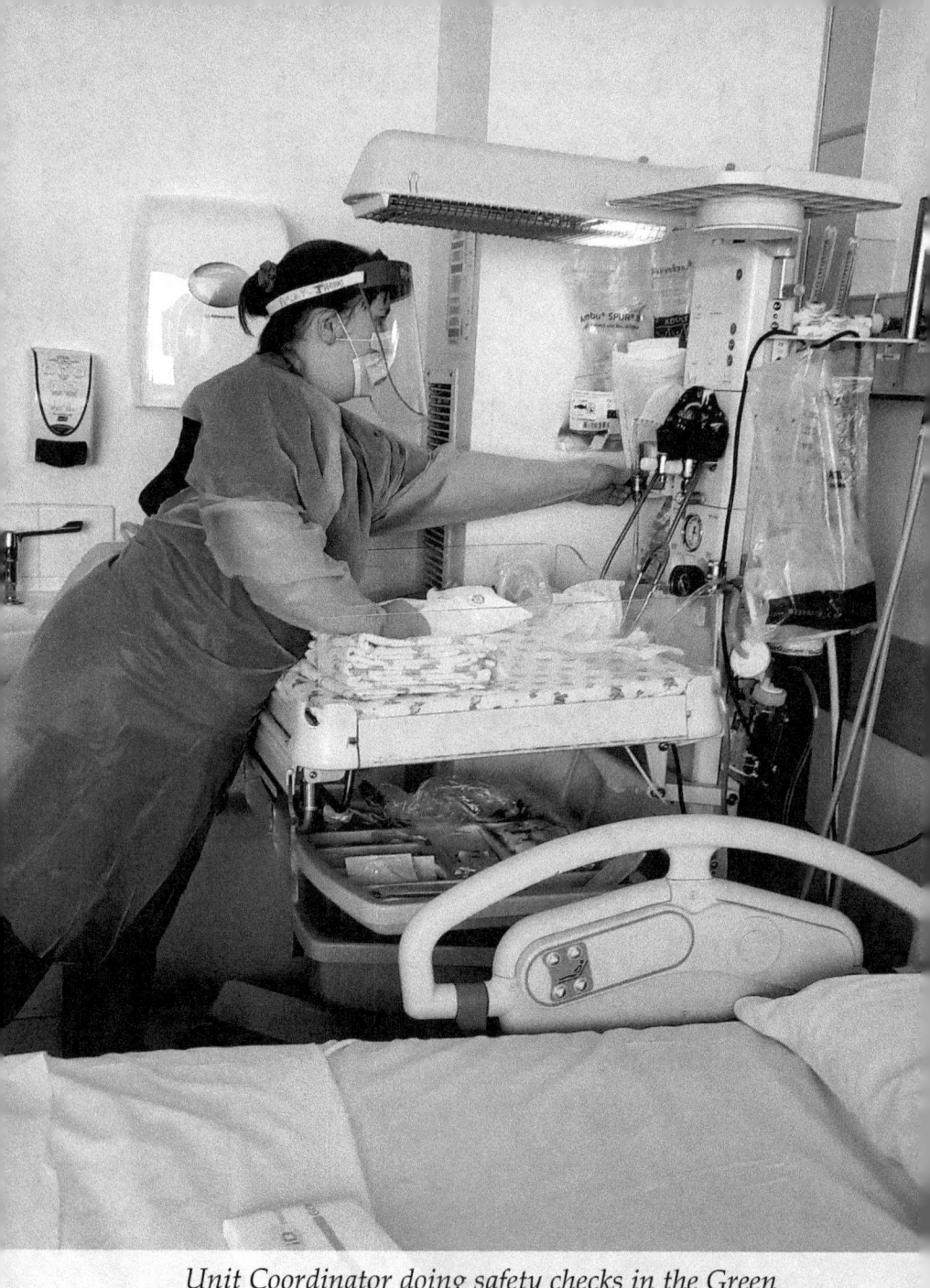

Unit Coordinator doing safety checks in the Green Zone Labour Ward

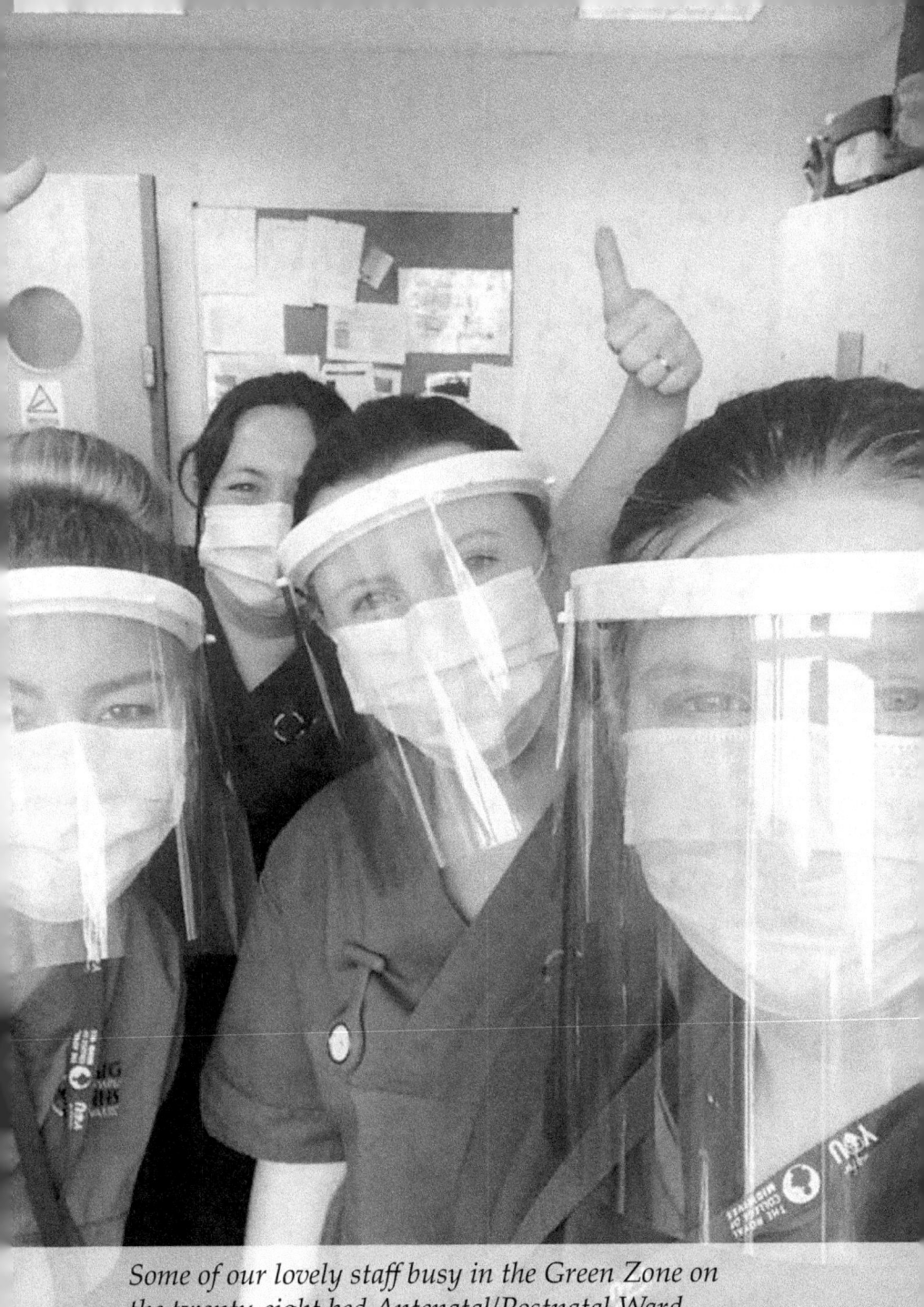
Some of our lovely staff busy in the Green Zone on the twenty-eight bed Antenatal/Postnatal Ward

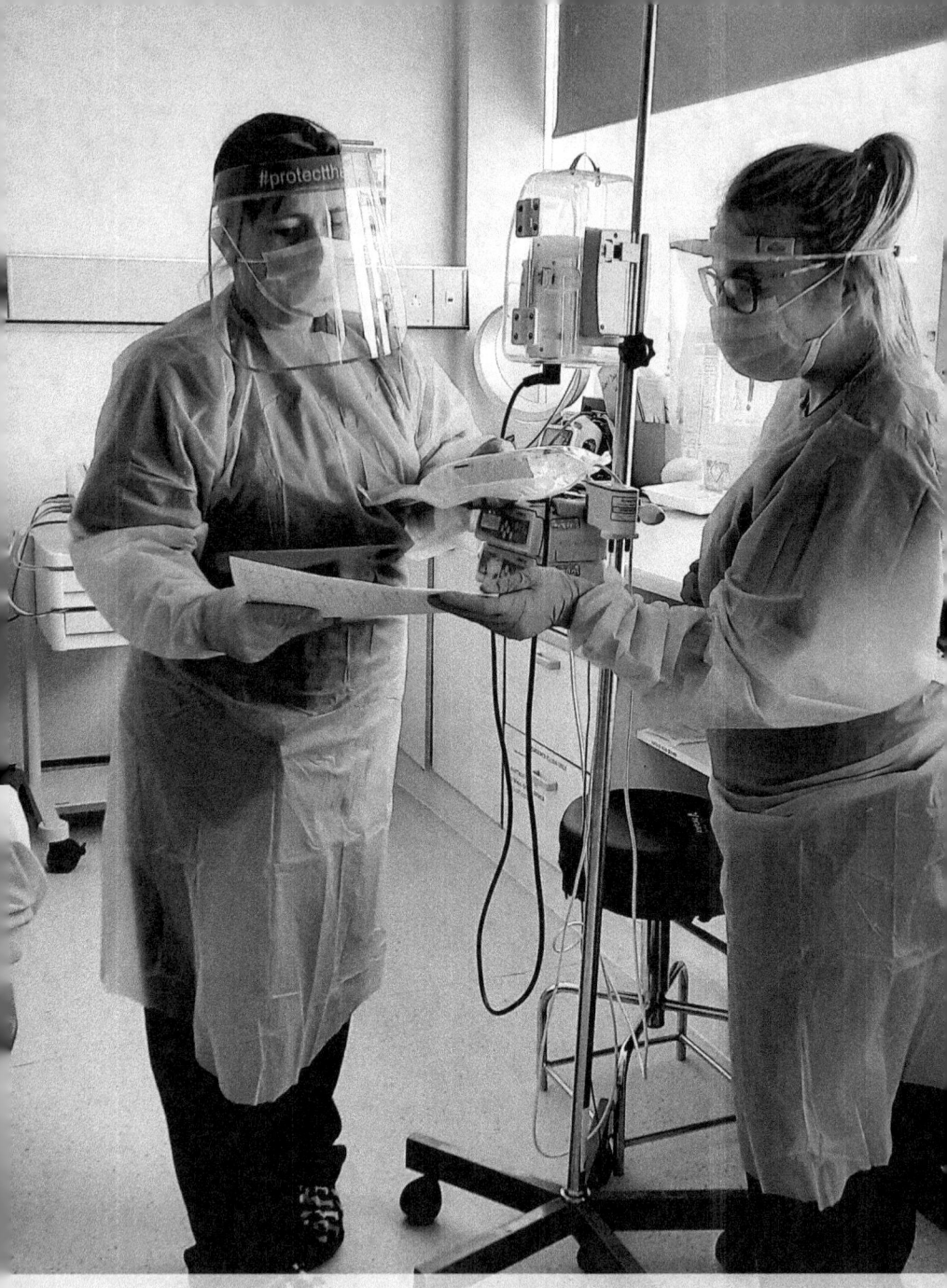

Checking medication together in Green Zone Labour Ward

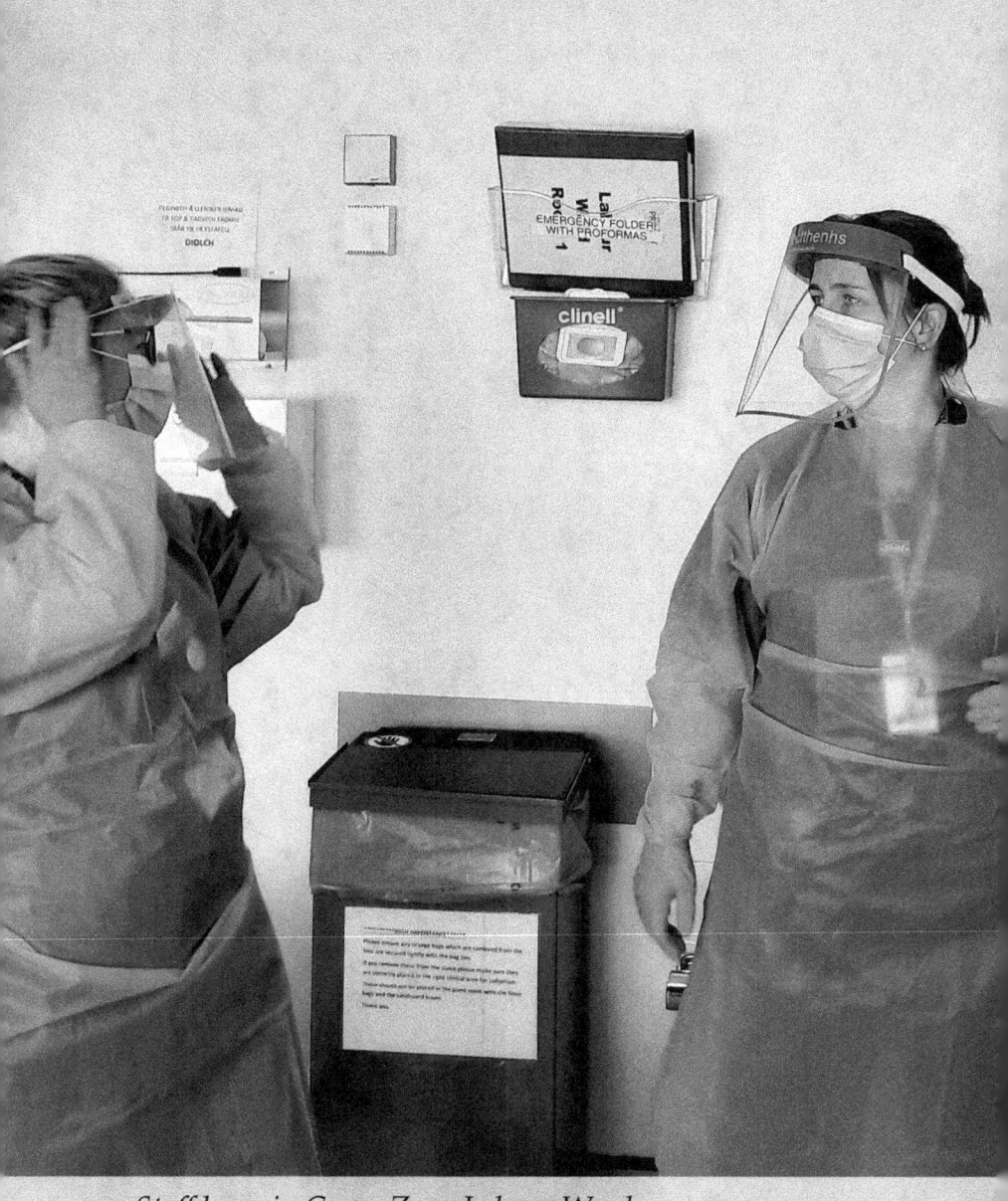
Staff busy in Green Zone Labour Ward

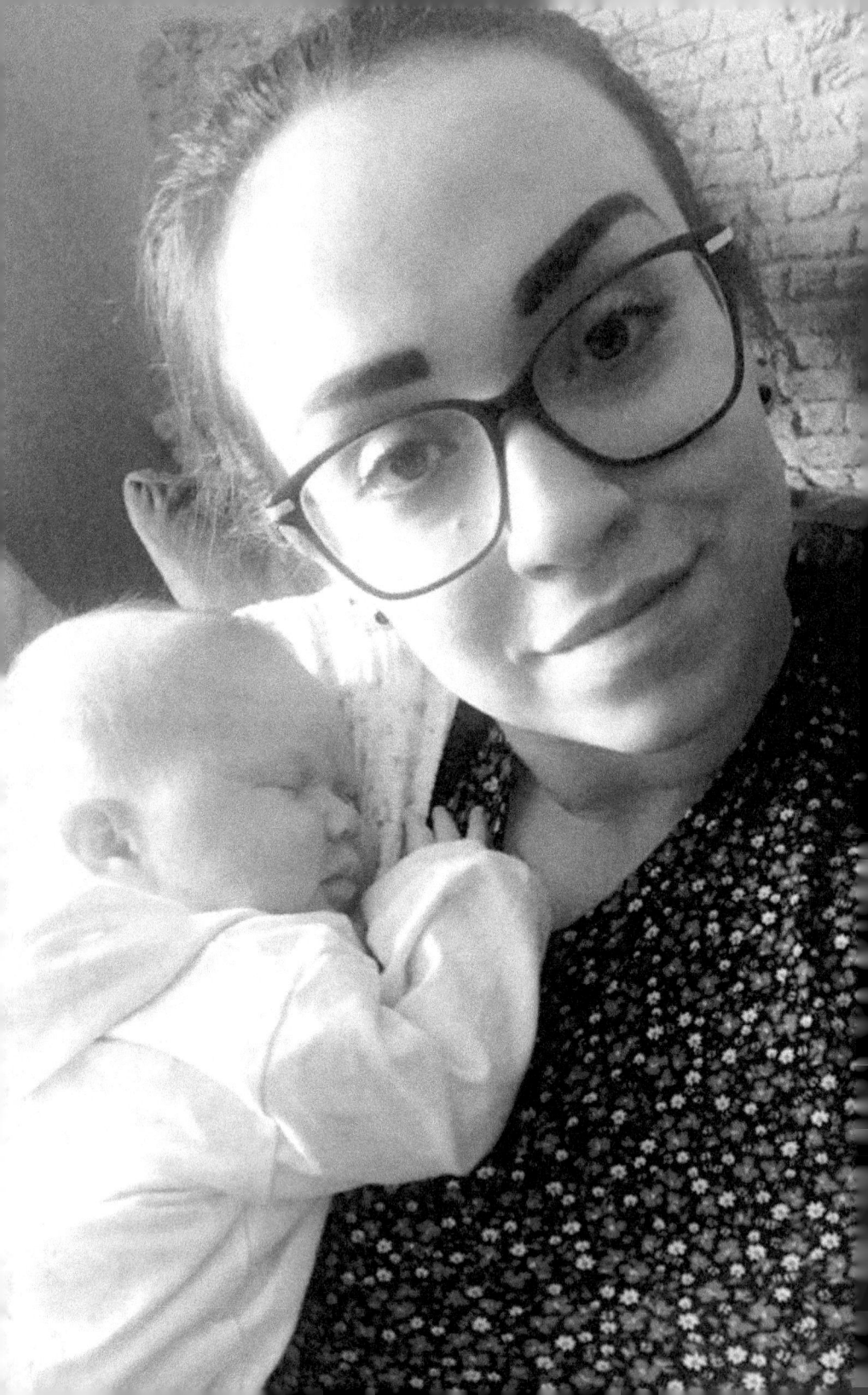

No. 1
Ffion's Story

When I found out I was pregnant, I was incredibly nervous for what the future held but thrilled at the same. I had done two-line tests and even though they both were showing positive results, I needed to confirm with a digital test for my own peace of mind. I remember having to call my best friend and get out of the house and go pick -up the test. My partner was working away at the time, but my news was very well appreciated!

I took me a while to accept that it was real after that. Even though I'd done the multiple tests and had the positive results it all still felt very surreal and I had experienced some bleeding at the beginning so that had sprung doubt into my mind. But I had a great support system in place between my best friend, her husband and my partner. We had told no one else straight away, we chose to wait until after the twelve-week scan.

After having confirmation that all was well with the baby and telling everyone about our news, I felt much better about everything and enjoyed my pregnancy. Even though it came with horrendous sickness and fatigue!

When it first came to light about the

coronavirus coming to the UK. I was worried and nervous about the uncertainty of it all, as most were, but didn't really think about the impact it would have on the final weeks of my pregnancy.

When the Prime Minister first announced that pregnant women can under the category of high risk I was 35 weeks at the time, my school that I work for were incredibly good and kept me at home for about a week before they began to shut. When lock down occurred that's when I really started to panic about my labour experience.

I still had a couple appointments to attend which felt strange because by this time, as measures had been put in place with regards to social distancing. I'd been stopped a couple times on route to the hospital by the police and queried on where I was headed, that used to make me rather flustered as even though I had a genuine reason to be out, I felt like I was being told off for being outside, I started to keep track on the many changes of rules about pregnancy in hospitals and that really made this nightmare a whole lot more real.

I had gone in to be induced on the 2nd of April at 9:00am due to my waters going at 37 weeks and within the space of half an hour of being there my partner had to leave as the rules had changed again and seeing him have to get up and walk away from me made me feel so vulnerable and alone. But the amazing Midwives did their upmost best to make me feel better about it all. I could text him throughout the day, but it wasn't the same. I had to ring him when I was heading down to the labour ward At 6pm which was I was told about maybe 5-10 minutes prior which made my partner anxious because he'd had to go home to wait and was factoring in the timeframe he had to get to me.

When down at the labour ward the Midwives I had were beyond amazing. They were so kind and friendly; they gave me a run down on everything available to me and made me feel so comfortable and relaxed. As the night and then morning went on, I wasn't progressing like I should of and got stuck at 4cm dilated. I ended up delivering by an emergency caesarean section, and that was very surreal, I felt very much defeated when that was mentioned, I had tried at labour for so long, drugged up and my body couldn't take it. I was rather frightened. I had never had any form of surgery before, though the surgeon and their team were beyond amazing. Laying on that table I can remember anxiously waiting to hear a cry and wondering how I'd feel? It felt like a lifetime and then when I heard it, I felt a release of built up anxiety. She was here, and she was safe.

Being at home has been strange. I haven't had

my parents fussing over my daughter or my siblings to visit, as everyone is in isolation. I haven't been able to show my daughter off to any of our family And Friends, it's been really hard. And now with my partner returning to work I sometimes feel lonely. But it's getting easier day by day.

Ffion's Story

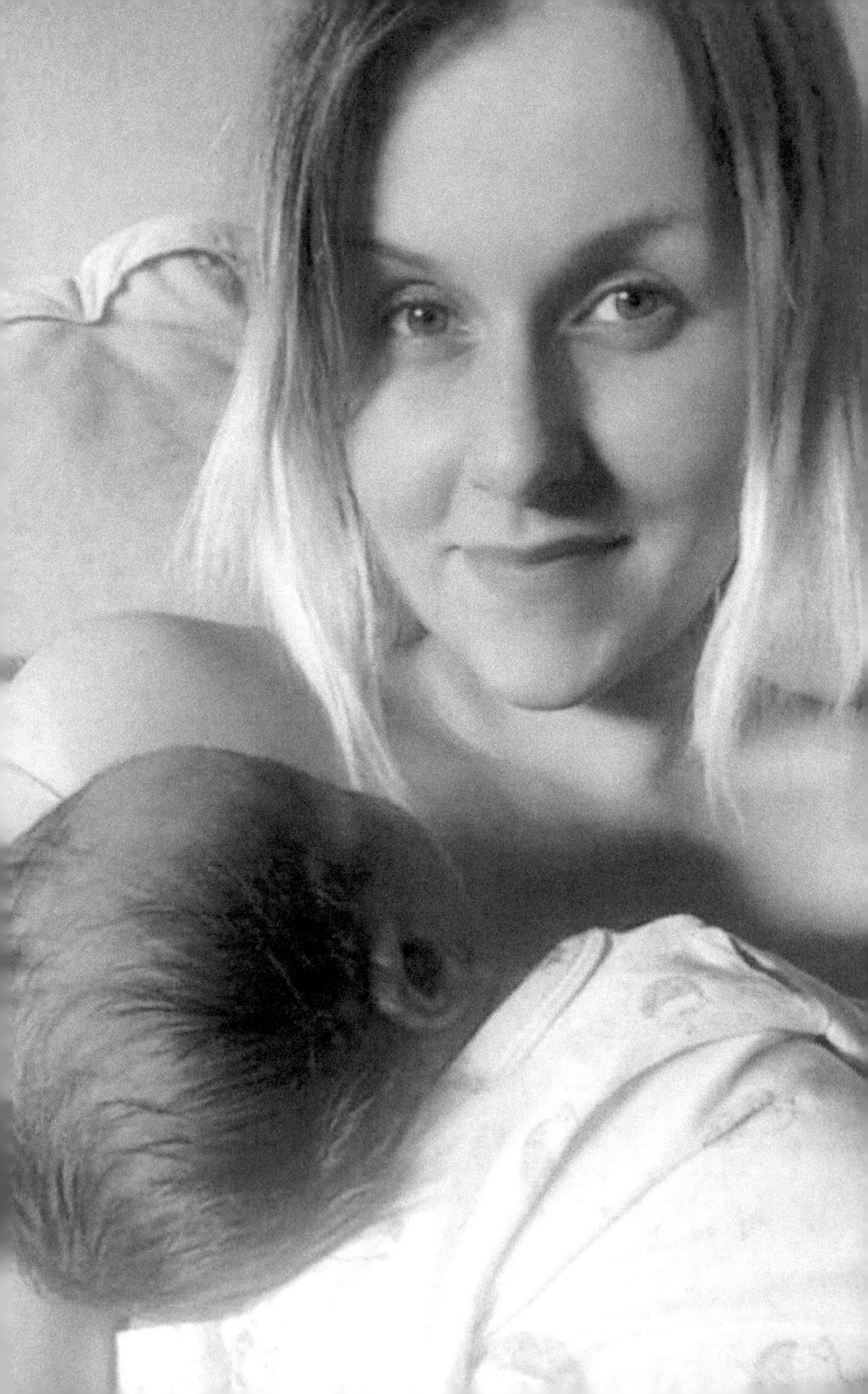

No. 2

Amy's Story

My little boy was born in Glangwili Hospital in early April. It's my second baby to be delivered in Glangwili Hospital and I wanted to share my experience to reassure any mums to be who may be concerned about giving birth in the hospital during the Covid-19 pandemic. Under the amazing care of the Glangwili Midwives and with the safety measures taken by the hospital, my birth and hospital stay were calm and controlled and at no point did I feel unsafe.

I was induced at exactly 40 weeks due to some abdominal pain that couldn't be pinpointed. Going into the hospital I was pleasantly surprised by how calm the ward was and to still see a smile on the faces of every Midwife I saw. There were fewer mums on the ward which meant apart from the necessary interaction with Midwives, I still felt safely distanced from other people and the wonderful level of individual care was not affected by the current health situation.

I was taken up to the labour ward after six hours of induction. The incredible Midwife who stayed with me throughout my labour knew I would not be able to have my husband there as he was looking after our little girl and she did not leave my side. Our little boy was born at 8lb 12oz after four long hours of pushing. I couldn't have gotten through without the amazing Midwife who supported me, and the exceptional care I received throughout my time in hospital.

Having had both my children in Glangwili Hospital, I have nothing but admiration and respect for the wonderful Midwives who have cared for both my children and brought them safely into the world. In amongst a frightening health situation, my experience was only of the calm and caring manner of every member of staff throughout each part of the hospital. Our midwives are incredible people who are working endlessly to keep us and our babies safe. Thank you to all the amazing staff at Glangwili and I hope my birth story helps mums out there who are worried about delivery at these difficult times. Trust our Midwives and trust out NHS.

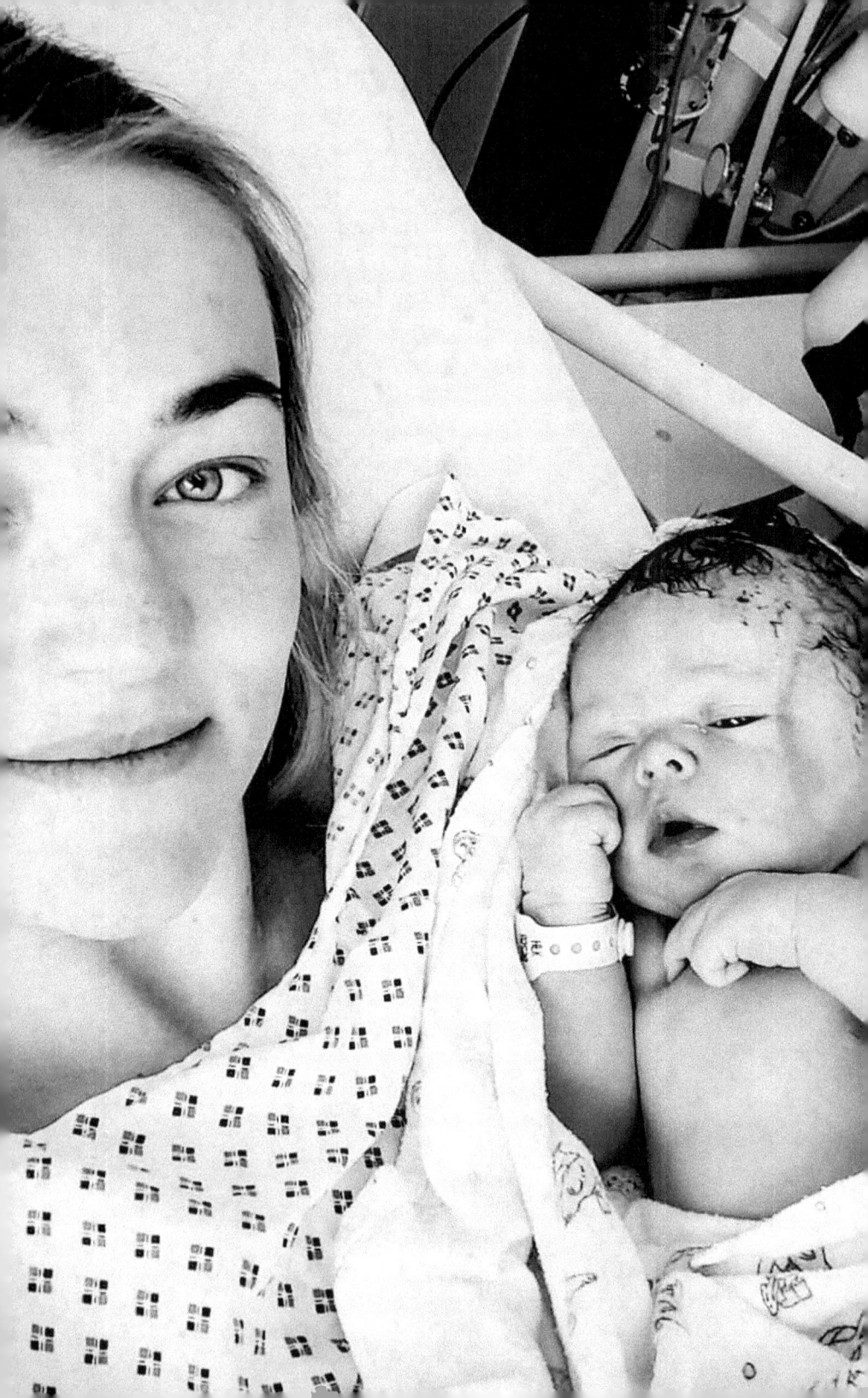

No. 3
Lucy's Story

The Midwife Led Unit was closed but I was in a room by myself in the Antenatal ward and I had two amazing Midwives that didn't leave my side. My labour was only 4 hours and 32 minutes and I was just on gas and air. It could have been a dream birth up until the final moment. Nancy's heartbeat started to drop because her head just couldn't get through, so I was taken to theatre and had an epidural straight away. There were around ten staff in theatre, and they all introduced themselves and were frankly the most amazing people I have ever met. I had an episiotomy and after two contractions thankfully my daughter was born on the second contraction. The team in theatre would have let me try to push once more and then it would have been an emergency section. They were all prepared from the minute I arrived in theatre and they were completely calm and supportive through it all.

Once finished in theatre, I had a Midwife and my mum, (my husband is in the shielding category so shared a virtual labour) with me in my own room for a few hours. They then took me up to the ward, where I stayed until I came home the next day. There are absolutely no visitors on the ward at all but again, the Midwives, Doctors and Health care assistants there all deserve medals. They cannot do enough for you.

For the time I stayed in the hospital I was in this perfect baby bubble, and it was as if coronavirus didn't even exist.
Glangwili is not what I thought it would be, or scary in anyway. The staff who helped me over those two days made this mad, scary world completely disappear, it was just about me and her.

My journey didn't end there. Once home, I began feeling better and better every day until Saturday afternoon. On the Saturday night I was admitted back into Glangwili Hospital with a temperature of 39.6. I got taken to the covid unit and put in a room by myself, Nancy joined me Sunday morning, she had to stay with my mum Saturday night while the incredible team of staff stabilised me. I was in that room until 6pm Monday night. They put me on Intra venous antibiotics straight away because my temperature had risen to 40.1 and they tested me for Covid. Sunday afternoon I also underwent a procedure to remove some stitches to try and take away some of the pressure-which thankfully did the trick and confirmed that everything was healing really well.

At 5pm Sunday, my temperature had been stable for 24 hours, my infection markers had come down and the call came from Cardiff to say I am covid free. With this news, my Husband was then able to come and pick his girls up, and we are now home as a family of three. I am telling you this because I have really been to hell and back the last few days but, yet again Glangwili Hospital Midwives and Doctors have literally saved me. Their unconditional dedication, support and commitment was next to none. The precautions in place are so rigorous and the constant encouragement from the staff there is endless.

From the bottom of mine and my family's hearts, Thank you. We owe you mine and my daughter's lives.

Birth Story

No. 4
Anonymous

Since the birth of my first child seven years ago, my periods have been fairly erratic. Even so, ten weeks was a long time, so I did a pregnancy test, but we had no way of working out how many weeks I was. After two early dating scans, we had a date for eight months later.

Since our Community Midwife came and completed the booking appointment at home in August, they have supported us every step of the way. I have Haemochromatosis and have a family history of Type 2 Diabetes and tested positive for Group B Strep early in the pregnancy. This meant that I was referred for consultant led care for labour, as we knew that I would need IV antibiotics because of the Strep-B.

I'm a runner, and in October, at 13 weeks, I put my trainers on the start line of the Cardiff Half. Despite taking it easy, I completed the course in under two hours. I continued running (but not racing) until mid-January.

By November, my baby had definitely settled into a pattern of movement. Then, one evening, we realised that my stomach was hard, and we'd not felt the usual movement pattern. A phone call later, and we were on our way to the hospital to be checked. We got home at 1am, happy that there was nothing wrong with the baby.

In January, we started thinking about the birth. We were told that due to the IV antibiotics, I would be unable to have a water birth, and that I would need to go to the ward as they were unable to administer the antibiotics at home.

In February, we attended the antenatal classes led by the Community Midwives. These were the last face to face classes they held. As covid-19 increasingly became part of our daily lives, the Midwives moved to You Tube. Whilst not the same as the face to face classes, being able to access the videos, and re-watch some of them (the yoga and breastfeeding ones especially) has been useful, but they don't replace the support you get at the face to face groups.

By the time we came to write the birth plan, at 36 weeks (early March) the social distancing guidelines were in place. I drove myself to the hospital, on my own, for the first time. Partners were no longer allowed to attend antenatal appointments with us. My Midwife was understanding and helpful. After completing the monitoring checks, we phoned my partner at home, put him on speaker phone, and completed my birth plan together. Whilst not what we had expected, it still allowed both of us to be part of the discussion and ask questions.

As I have a 7-year old, childcare was a serious consideration for labour and birth. The original plan had my Mam moving to stay at her caravan, five minutes from our house, from 39 weeks. This would have given us childcare and help after birth should I need a Caesarean section. Covid meant this was no longer an option, and we had to have a rapid rethink.

As we headed towards the due date, the updates to policy and guidelines posted in the Facebook group became more frequent. My partner and I started planning, and mentally preparing for the fact that I might have to give birth without him. Either because it was no longer allowed, or because we had no other child care options at short notice. The stress got to me; my partner concerned that I might sink into the depression that first reared its head after the birth of my daughter.

We contacted my daughter's Dad. We are relatively fortunate in that her Dad is working from home, and the guidelines allowed for children under eighteen to travel between parents' homes. This meant that we were able to treat the two houses as one as there was no contact outside the four of us. Thankfully, he was prepared to be our childcare, whatever time of day we needed him. My partner works for the NHS. My daughter's Dad has allowed the back and forth to continue, despite this putting him (and our daughter) at a higher risk than would otherwise be the case.

The remainder of my antenatal appointments were during lockdown. the hospital was strangely quiet, but, with the exception of the fact that my partner couldn't attend with me, they continued as normal. We opted to discontinue extra scans in order to decrease the number of visits and the amount of time spent at the hospital.

On 14th April, my waters broke after lunch with a long slow continuous trickle. We phoned the hospital, and my partner and my daughter took me to the ward, waved goodbye at the door at 2:30pm, and went home. Partners were no longer allowed until active labour, and my daughter wouldn't get to see me or meet her sister until we were home again. We contacted my daughter's Dad to let him know that I was in hospital, and that we would be in contact with him again once we knew when my partner needed to come to the hospital.

There was minimal interaction with the ward staff. No chats, and no laughing like there had been for my first.

Early evening, the midwives started the IV, and my contractions were stronger and closer together. At 7:30pm, my daughter phoned to say goodnight. At 10:30pm, the Midwife told me to phone my partner and tell him to make his way to the hospital. My partner phoned my little girl's Dad, woke her up, dropped her off, and came to the hospital.

I was in labour overnight, and increasingly tired. We walked, we spent time in the bath, spent ages in the shower. In the early hours of the morning, totally exhausted, I had pethidine and I managed to sleep for a while. I woke up around 5:30am, with my partner calling for the Midwives as I was calling out in my sleep. As they arrived, I felt the need to push.

The Midwife wore PPE, including a visor, full apron and a mask. After getting stuck in the birth canal, narrowly avoiding a last-minute emergency caesarean section, an hour and a half later, my daughter was born. I lost a lot of blood. Once we were moved to the Postnatal Ward, my partner was asked to leave.

I stayed in hospital with my baby girl overnight as we both had to be monitored. No visitors were allowed. My 7-year-old video called from her Dad's to see her sister. My partner called and video- called throughout the day. My haemoglobin levels were low, and I needed iron tablets before I could go home. It was lonely. I am so glad we packed my kindle and were able to see each other.

The following morning, the Health care support worker collected the iron tablets and we called my partner to come to collect us. He brought the car seat to the door of the ward, but wasn't allowed in. The Midwives carried my Daughter and the bags to the door.

Post-natal home visits were made by my Midwife. But all discussion was completed over the phone before they arrived. She spent as little time as possible in the house. Before entering, she had to don her PPE. Apron, gloves, goggles and mask in the street outside. It was all a bit surreal. The Midwifery and Obstetric teams at Bronglais were brilliant. The information and support they provided was essential in making a difficult time less stressful than it might have been.

We aren't able to register her birth. We can't get that all important piece of paperwork that opens so many other doors ... Passports, bank accounts. Even registering her with the GP is more complex than usual as only the Health Visitors are able to complete the registration forms.

But there is no doubt that there is a feeling of lost time, because my maternity leave has a finite end date. There is a chance that my baby girl will never get to experience mother and toddler groups, not see another baby, before I have to go back to work.

The fun bits of getting ready for a newborn, and her early months have been taken from us ... we never finished the shopping before lockdown, now we're struggling to get clothes in small baby sizes. The buggy is still at my parents' house in South Wales.

There have been advantages, the lockdown has meant that we have been able to settle into a routine for us. The lack of visitors is hard in some respects, we don't know when the grandparents will be able to meet their granddaughter and give her cwtches, we haven't been able to meet our newborn niece who lives in London. In others, it has been a revelation. No visitors meant no constant interruptions, and feeding has been easier to establish. No school runs meant we've been able to adapt our routine around the baby's needs, without making my 7-year-old feel like she's an inconvenience.

My partner, still working, is doing shifts in blocks. This makes it easier for him to keep away from his newborn daughter for a block of time, and then come home. At some point, if he is reassigned, we know he will have to move out to protect all of us. Neither of us is looking forwards to that, but minimising the risks has to come first.

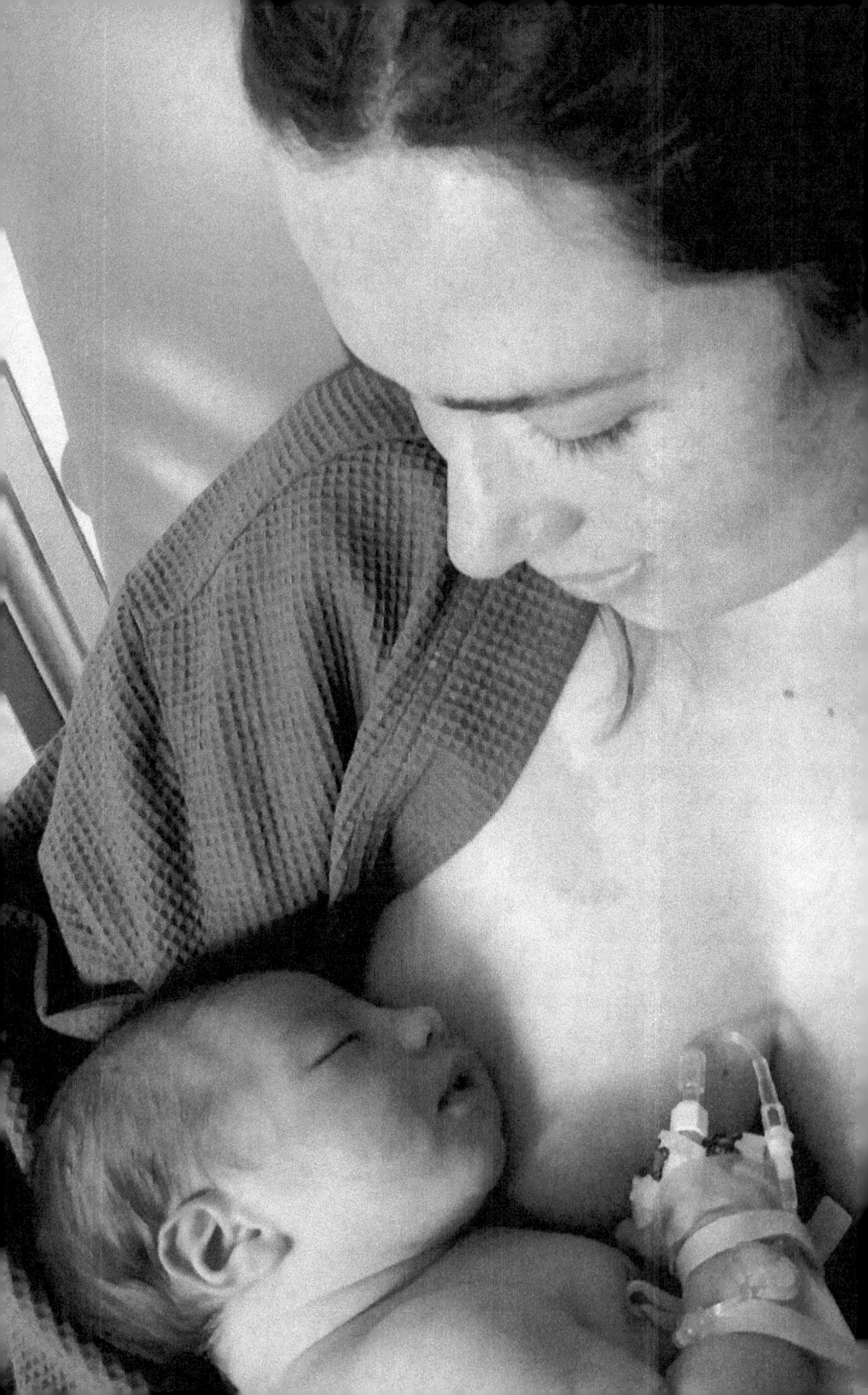

No. 5

Seren's Story

When I got pregnant, I dearly hoped to have a normal birth (VBAC- Vaginal birth after caesarean section) this time after a previous unplanned caesarean section due to slow progress (aka 'failure to progress'). I am still shocked and elated to say that it happened for me. From my perspective on both experiences all I can say is, that all births are epic journeys, and all mothers are warriors however they birth, and each birth was a personal Everest for me.

This birth was also during April 2020 in the covid 19 pandemic. Apart from the concerns about how changing protocols might affect my birth choices the real challenges during my labour were the existing triggers relating to my previous birth, i.e. the physical restrictions of continuous monitoring, the fear being 'on the clock' and facing the possibility of another caesarean section.

There were many hurdles to cross to get to our normal birth, starting before the birth, from the psychological challenge of revisiting and unravelling the previous birth story, to the endless weeks of breech presentation, making peace with the decision to go for an elective if the baby didn't turn (which he did at the

11th hour), then going overdue and heading for induction. Ever since my first birth when I heard of friends having a natural delivery, I would be relieved and very happy for them, then quietly shed a tear for me and my birth. I had to be careful not to ride the wave of other people's stories online in the run up to my birth. It felt like a massive test of my ability to trust and surrender.

After self-isolating for two weeks even ahead of lockdown as a precaution I went 10 days overdue and careered towards induction. I really wanted a spontaneous labour to improve chances of a normal birth. However, after a moonlit walk and a relaxing 'last' date night I went into spontaneous labour on the morning of induction. Luckily, my mum had isolated with us and could take our eldest. We laboured at home for nine hours using breathing and music for a beautiful oxytocin fuelled early labour.

We called hospital once timings indicated active labour. On arrival my partner took me to the door of the Midwife Led Unit area where he had to wait outside in the car until I had been internally examined to confirm I was in active labour. Then he was phoned, had his temperature taken and could stay for the duration. He would not have been allowed to stay if he had a high temperature. The Midwives were all wearing gloves, mask and plastic aprons but their eyes and their words all conveyed reassurance, humanity and compassion.

We spent twelve hours in an Midwife Led Unit private room (not the usual Midwife Led Unit rooms which are now used for c0vid -19 and there are no birth pools) keeping up our good vibes and labouring with music, aromatherapy and up- breathing. We were given plenty of privacy and positive encouragement from a lovely Midwife and had use of a bath. Twelve hours in and having remained at 4cm dilated, we agreed to go to labour ward and break the waters. We walked to the ward, where our wishes for dimmed lighting and using our music were facilitated. Breaking the waters to speed things up which was a relief. I started using gas and air at this point in conjunction with up-breathing, it just felt like the right moment. This is also when I met my personal triggers; the continuous monitoring just didn't work, they slipped around, the scalp electrode didn't work. Finding myself confined to 2ft radius of the monitor and with the kind midwives kneeling and hovering around to keep the slippy monitors on I started to lose my ability to cope with intensifying surges. This is when I began to give up. I felt that after so many hours labouring and with a deadline of six hours from waters breaking to full dilation, I was set to fail. I began to say that if it was all due to end in caesarean-section again that I might as well call it a day. But the Midwives were saying that I was doing well, and it was my partner's encouragement to just do a bit longer that kept me going. He kept reminding me that it was when I wanted to give up that the miracle was about to happen. I realise now that this was probably also part of 'transition' as surges were coming thick and fast. He also voiced what I couldn't articulate, which was that I needed to try not having continuous monitoring. Freed from those constraints I was able to labour actively as I needed. We progressed quite quickly, and baby was born just under five hours after breaking the waters. Being told I could push at last was the most wonderful thing. Pushing and birthing my baby was a truly awesome, powerful experience.

The elation of birth was followed by a sort of empty shock as the baby required help to breath having swallowed meconium on arrival. A team of people appeared as if from nowhere to revive him. We saw him breathing and knew he would be ok, then he was taken to the Special Care Baby Unit. Sometime later my partner went to meet him for twenty minutes before having to go home. Then I was able to stay on Postnatal ward and visit him any time and establish feeding. My baby was back with me after about twenty -four hours to my eternal relief. The care and compassion shown to all of us was immense and I couldn't fault it, even as the staff were working in hot sweaty masks and gloves.

Days and nights on postnatal ward without visitors and no dads allowed was both a chance to rest and reflect in a kind of limbo land, and a challenge, taking care of a baby while recovering from birth. All mums were in separate rooms. The care on this ward was so very kind and gentle.

My birth with all its twists and turns was a very positive, healing experience. I have eternal gratitude to my partner and to all the staff at the hospital. I also had amazing phone support towards the end of the third trimester from a friend and Doula who's listening, witnessing, reflection and encouragement helped me to emotionally prepare. During labour we called her several times for support to make choices at critical moments. This additional perspective was a huge help and empowered my partner in supporting me and giving voice to my needs.

A note about after-care which is really important, but we often don't tend to think about it much before the birth- even more important with social distancing precluding your usual carousel of visitors- the nature of after-care contact is notably different due to covid 19. Much is being done on the phone wherever possible. I still had two house calls to help with breastfeeding during the two routine visits. But otherwise as much as possible is over the phone. I think this really requires mums to be proactive and pick up the phone if you have any concerns and ask for over the phone advice. I have done this for breastfeeding support, and I have friends who have needed to do this to keep an eye on potential infections. A stitch in time saves nine, don't suffer in silence, the support is still there, call before anything gets really bad!

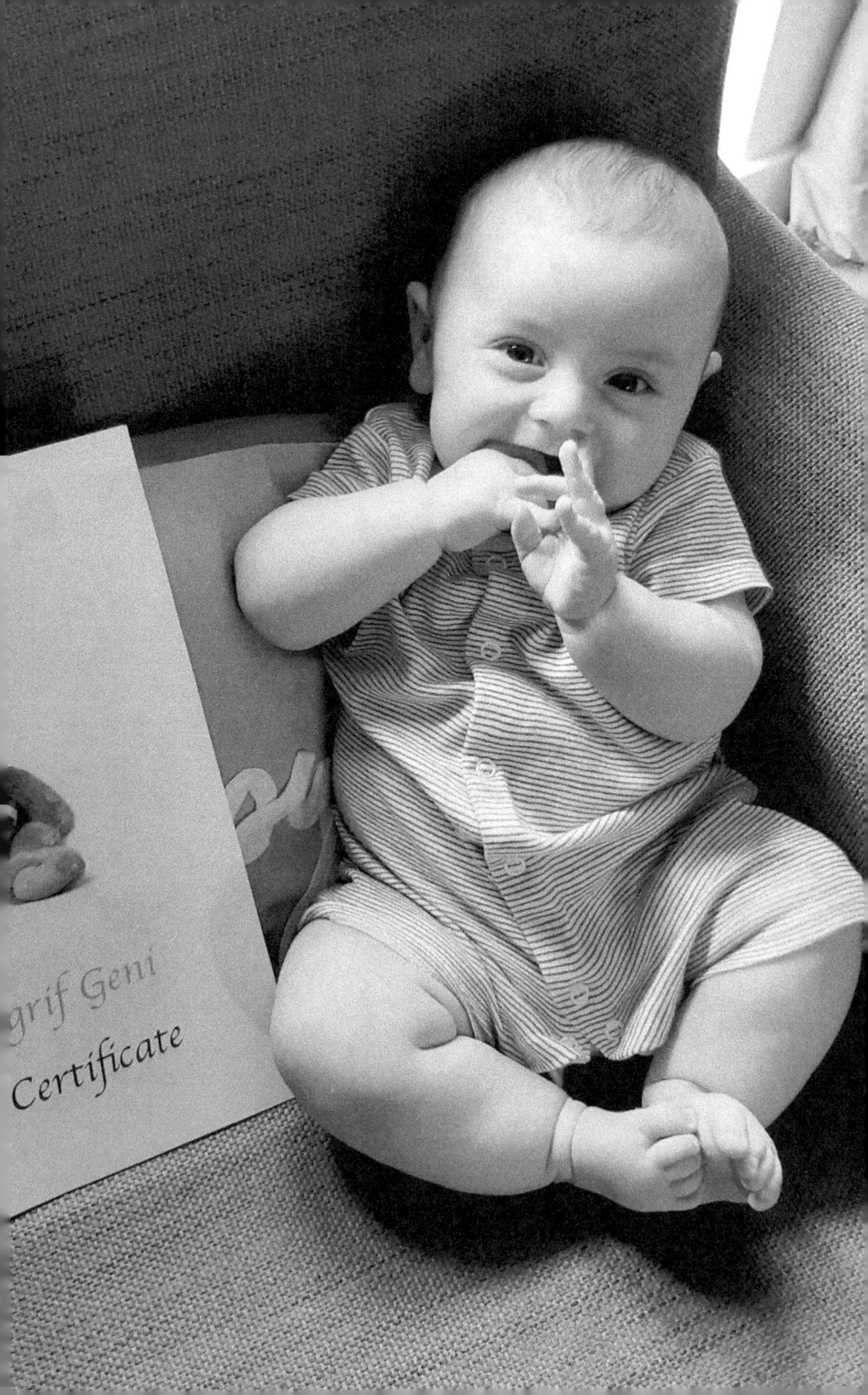

No. 6
Emma's Story

After trying for a baby for four years and losing four stone in weight, also having suffered a miscarriage five years ago, I was referred for investigations to double check that I was not suffering with polycystic ovarian syndrome (PCOS). This was done the middle of June 2019 and on the 7th August 2019, I found out I was seven weeks pregnant. I was very reluctant to do a test because I didn't want to be disappointed, again. We were both over the moon and it took weeks for the news to sink in.

I referred myself to the Midwives and was Consultant led from the beginning due to my high BMI. I was allocated a Midwife and she came to see me when I was ten weeks as I was due to go on holiday for fortnight. I think we both walked around in a haze, one of my holidays was a girl's holiday to Disney Land Paris for five days and I spent a large portion of that time sleeping as the first trimester wiped me out.

My pregnancy went well. We were told we were due on or around 8th April 2020. I would go as far as to say that I enjoyed it, the feeling of baby moving was something special. I was told that I had to have Clexane injections and take Aspirin daily to prevent any complications. I would have to have the glucose tolerance test and that was fine. The downs syndrome test came back as a high chance, I then had to have a further blood test, that was the worst two weeks of waiting. But all was fine.

As the pregnancy progressed, I had to have serial scans for sizing baby...every three weeks I attended Bronglais Hospital for a scan and then go to the antenatal clinic to see the Midwives and the Consultant. It always went smoothly and never had any problems. There were a few occasions where I had to attend the ward as baby's movements were either less than usual or a changed pattern. The care we received was outstanding and I couldn't fault it. We were always put at ease.

From the very beginning I wanted my husband and my mum in with me as birthing partners and we were all looking forward to that day.

I finished work on Thursday, 12th March, just as the world was shocked by the covid-19 outbreak. I work at a GP surgery locally so was relieved to say the least that I was now safe at home but still had freedom to see family and friends. On Fri, 13th March I had to go to an outpatients appointment with an Anaesthetist, this was to see whether they would be able to locate the right section of my spine to do an epidural if I needed a caesarean-section. They were happy this could be achieved, if it couldn't be (depending on the day) they would have to put me under general anaesthetic. I hoped this wouldn't have to happen and I would get the birth I wanted, within reason. A water birth with gas and air and my two nominated birthing partners. I should also mention that I had to have a meeting with Manual Handling staff at Bronglais, again, due to my BMI. Again, they were happy and didn't foresee any problems.

My penultimate scan at 36 weeks showed baby was 9lbs 6oz-ish and that was with four weeks to go. The Consultant wasn't too sure whether or not to book me for a further scan in three weeks, but thankfully she did. Importantly, my husband was still allowed to come with me to the appointments at this stage.

So, during the next three weeks I was busy cooking our "little" bundle of joy, not being able to drive as bump prevented me getting behind the wheel and the UK were bracing themselves for a pandemic and soon followed the announcement we were all dreading... we were put on lock down! I was faced with questions such as "Is my husband allowed to come to the appointments?", "Is my husband going to see our first child being born?" answers that would all soon come to light...

Now, I joined the bumps Facebook page to keep up to date with the ever-changing policies and guidance and the news I had been dreading, all expectant mothers had to attend their appointments on their own. I was due to attend for my last scan and on the 2nd April at 39+1 weeks pregnant and now waddling along I went to the appointment on my own, having had a lift from my Dad. My scan went well, then I was told baby was likely to be 11lbs 8oz to which my eyes watered but I took it in my stride and thought "I can handle this, my body will only grow a baby I am capable of carrying and birthing". Hmmm... they would be my famous last words. Off I went to the antenatal clinic, there I discovered that my blood pressure was higher than normal and the Consultant told me that I would never be able to birth the baby naturally, I needed to go to the ward and speak to the consultant on duty and book in for a caesarean-section. He also mentioned that I may not be able to have the baby at Bronglais Hospital and might have to go to Glangwili Hospital. I did not want this to happen, I was shocked to say the least but trundling up the corridor I called my Dad and told him to go home, and I would call when I am done.

Once on the ward I was looked after by a Midwife that I had not met before, but she did an excellent job of talking me through everything, calming me down and giving advice. There I met the Consultant who came in to talk me through the pros and cons of both options (natural and caesarean section). I decided, once I got over the shock that the best and safest option for me was to have a caesarean section. It all went quite quickly from there, a Doctor came in to go through the consent form and I was worried about healing after the operation as I have an apron already and wanted to make sure this wouldn't cause problems. Everyone reassured me that with care and attention it would be okay. I also, in my 31 years have never had surgery before so having any form of anaesthetic and going under the knife was daunting. I then thought it best to ask when I would be having said baby, and it just so happened that they had a slot the following day and there it was, I was told to go home and come back at 8am having taken the omeprazole given to me and nil by mouth after 10pm. It is also important to point out that my blood pressure had gone down and they were happy to go ahead with everything.

Off home I went, I was in shock that we were going to have our baby the following day. I was nervous so didn't sleep much that night and had been awake since 4am working out whether we had everything ready, did I have everything I needed in my hospital bag and stuff for baby. I sat and watched my husband have breakfast whilst I sipped water and then the time came to go to hospital. My husband was allowed to come with me and could stay for the birth, we were looked after really well.

I can't put into words how relaxed I felt, and they helped to put my husband at ease. We were talked through everything and told that I was second on the list.

We eventually made the journey down to theatre and I was wheeled in to see the Anaesthetist and my husband was told to wait until someone came out to get him. Unless there was a problem with the epidural and I had to have general anaesthetic. Time was getting on, but on the second attempt and with a lot of breathing exercises and support they eventually managed it and everything else happened in a flash. My husband was bought in to the theatre and sat next to me awaiting the news. I heard the Consultant call for forceps and imagined baby was probably the size that they estimated, if not slightly bigger.

Eventually, there was the long-awaited cry and the Midwife popped around the screen and introduced us to our son. He was (and is) perfection. All the theatre staff and those that were in recovery were marvellous. There was no talk of the coronavirus, everyone got on with their jobs and made us feel at ease.

After my short stop in recovery back we went to the ward. Our baby boy was weighed and was a whopping 10lbs 13oz. It wasn't long before my legs regained feeling and the Midwives wanted me up on my feet, I was happy to try this. I wanted to get on with recovery as soon as possible. My husband was allowed to stay with us until 8pm. We were moved to our own room and once we were settled, he had to leave. The hardest part was knowing that he was not allowed back in the following day and if I was to stay in an extra night it would be just me and the little one. That night I made every effort to get myself out of bed and to the toilet, it was uncomfortable to say the least. The Midwives and Health Care Assistants were marvellous, they came every time I pressed the buzzer and helped me with baby and were very good at telling me that I was doing a fantastic job and taking it all in my stride. I needed the encouragement.

Saturday morning came and I was excited to go home and finally be a family. My plans were put on hold as I was not walking very well and on discussing my going home with one of the Midwives to whom I would be forever grateful for, I came to realise that I would need to get up the stairs, use the toilet as the toilets in the hospital are higher up. I was upset as I wanted to see my husband, and also wanted my husband to spend more time with his son. A few phone calls, a few tissues and pain relief later I agreed it was in fact the best thing for both of us to stay in an extra night. I was helped to the shower and left alone with my son for a few hours to get some sleep, and I felt better. The plan was to go home around 11.00am on the Sunday.

Sunday morning came and I woke feeling better than I did the day before. The Consultant and another Doctor came to see me and talk me through the operation. All went well, no problems. I had the "you should lose weight" conversation, contraception and other information. They checked my wound, twenty-two staples I had and to be fair I had no problems and the wound was really good, everyone was happy. I was nearly set to leave; I had breakfast and went for a shower then phoned my husband to come and get us. He was not allowed back onto the ward, so he had to bring the pram and car seat to the door and a Midwife bought it to me to put baby in.

Getting into the car was an adventure but after a good five-minute attempt I managed it. After a ten-minute journey we were home.

My mum and Dad had made us a Sunday dinner, so they came over and delivered that. They only saw the baby from a distance.

We are now four weeks down the line and it is very, very hard being new parents and you can't even see your family or friends and they all feel the same. Both me and baby were discharged by our Community Midwife two weeks after we left hospital as my wound was healing well and baby was back over his birth weight. We have had contact from the Health Visitor, only via telephone and then appointment for baby's immunisations at the end of May. So, despite all this and the sleepless nights I am going to say we are doing a good job without the "normal" support network.

The coronavirus could not have come at a more inconvenient time for us, but we are in our bubble and we are safe.

We as a family will be forever grateful to the Community Midwives, the Antenatal clinic staff, Gwenllian ward staff and Consultants, Doctors and the whole Theatre team as well as the Sonographers for all their care and attention during the last nine months and for bringing our beautiful baby boy into the world, safe and sound.

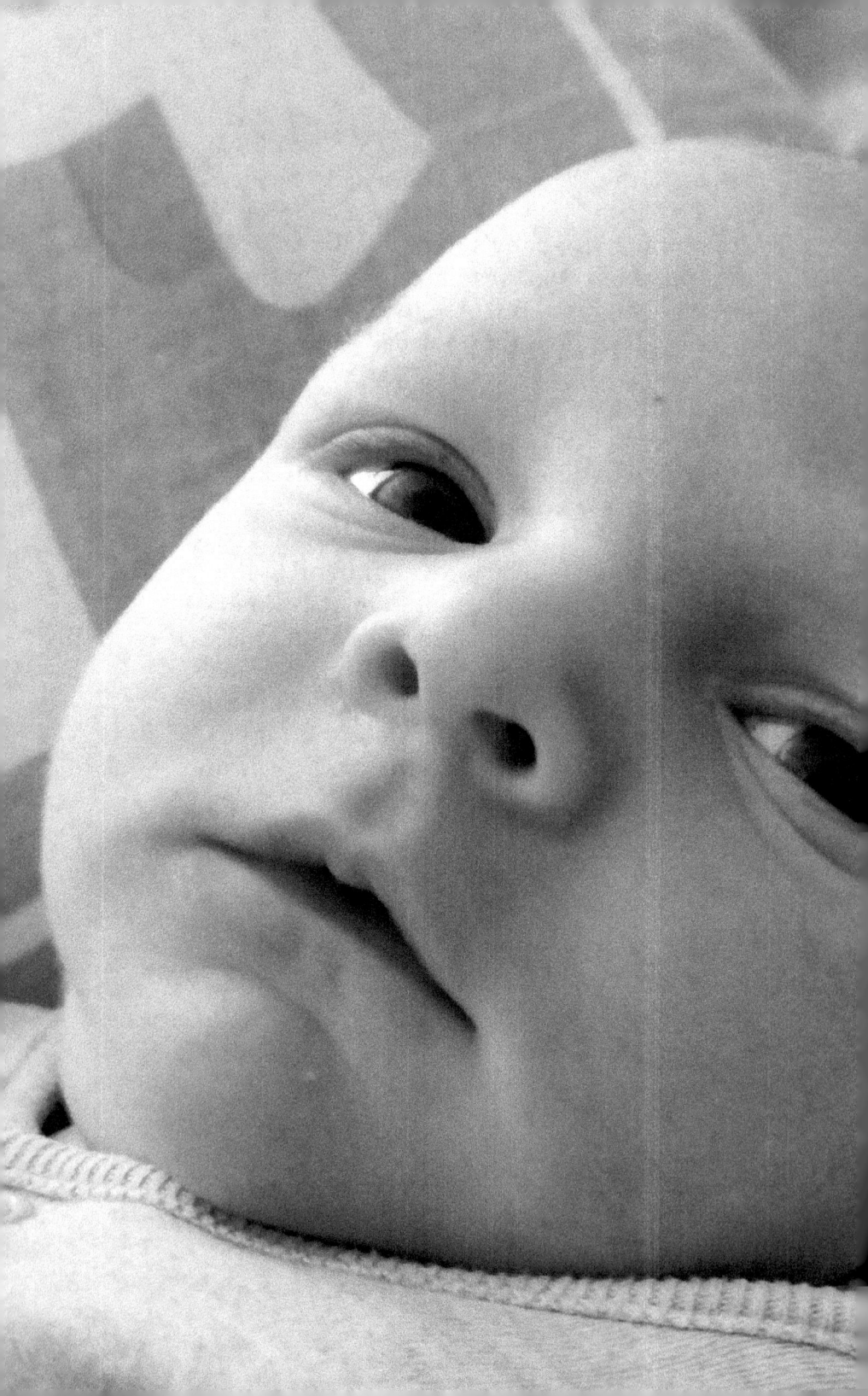

No. 7
Eleri's Story

Our second son was born via elected caesarean section on Friday 20th March which was the Friday before lockdown was declared. The staff on the ward were absolutely amazing at putting my mind at ease as I suffer with anxiety. They reassured me constantly and made me feel at ease throughout. The Midwives, Doctors and Health care support workers were very supportive and made my stay more bearable. Although currently I am suffering with anxiety, I know that Gwenllian Ward are only a phone call away if I need reassurance at any time of day or night. This also goes to my Community Midwife whom I would like to thank from the bottom of my heart. She's always a text away if I need some advice.

It was only during the end of my pregnancy that the covid-19 became apparent. I visited my pre op appointment on my own and felt very nervous. I didn't need to though as the ward staff were reassuring and welcoming.

I am at the moment just taking one day at a time because if I think too far ahead it sends my anxiety through the roof. I'm finding it difficult without family and friends but am very grateful that I have a supportive partner and two gorgeous boys.

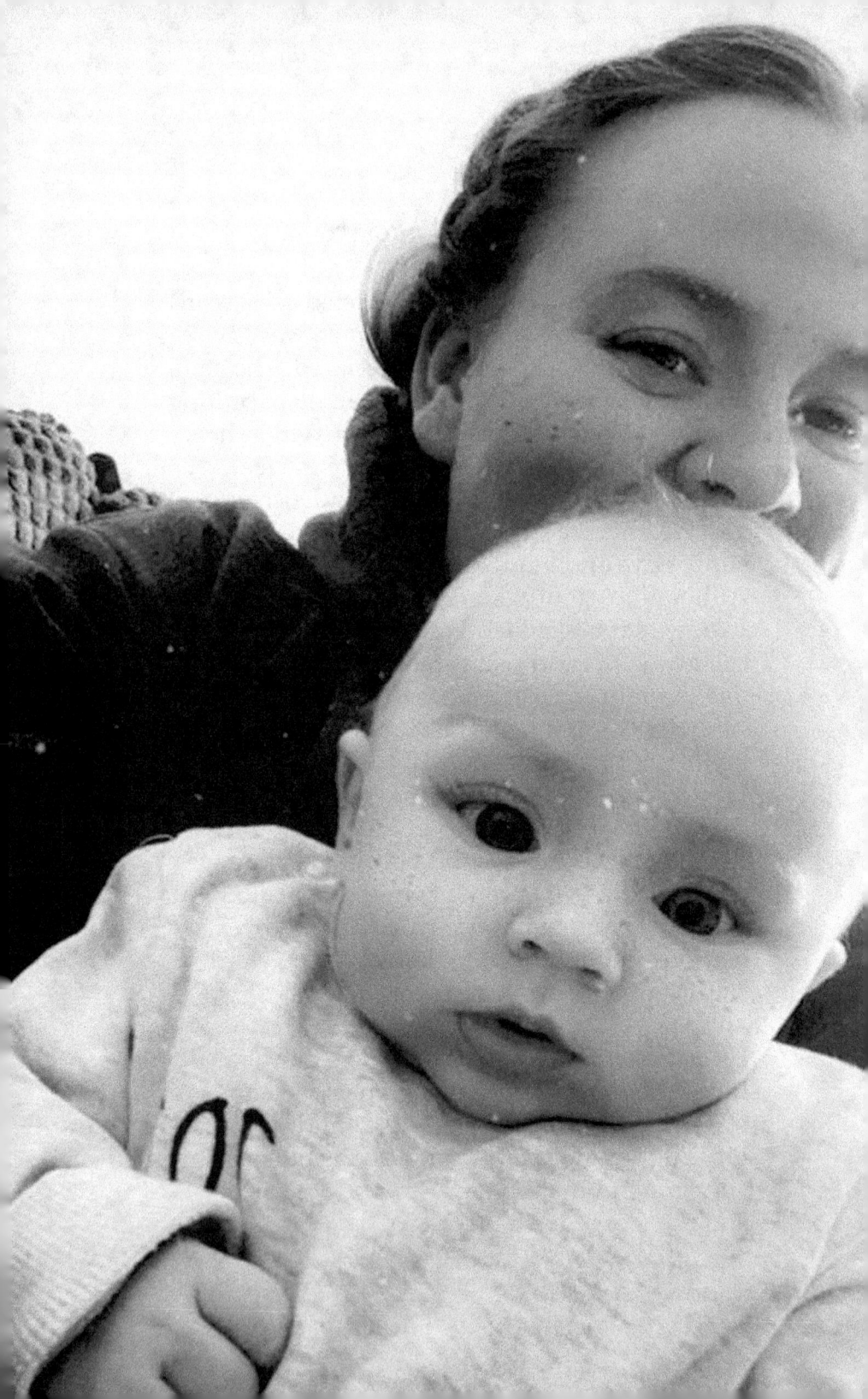

No. 8

Natasha's Story

So, when I found out I was pregnant me and my partner weren't actually together, we made the decision to try and make it work after finding out we were having another baby.
I can't say I was shocked to find out I was pregnant, me and my partner weren't exactly being careful and I hadn't been on birth control for nearly two years before falling pregnant, our view was we've been together five years of – 'if it happens it happens'.

Since this coronavirus has taken over it's been quite difficult, more so for my partner, who had been very hands on during the pregnancy. So, for him not to be able to come to anymore antenatal appointments was hard. I found myself being judged a lot while I was pregnant during this pandemic more so for the fact that I still had to go out and do the shopping, I found that people were staring.

My Baby was born on the 7th of April. I went into labour at 1am on the 7th and phoned the hospital at 3.30am, upon reaching the hospital at 4.30am I was examined and found to be 4cm which enabled my partner to come into the delivery room with me straight away, which proved it was worth waiting to go into hospital.

The Midwives were absolutely amazing throughout my labour, the labour ward was very relaxed, they listened to all of my requests and did their best to fulfil them. My daughter finally arrived at 12.14 on the 7th of April weighing 6lb 1.5oz. After two hours with Dad we were taken down to ward and dad left, I think that was the only disappointment out of the whole experience was that we didn't get a lot of time for Dad to bond with our Baby, while I can appreciate why Dad couldn't stay it was probably the hardest thing of the whole labour was knowing that he would have to go home to Milford Haven while I was in Carmarthen.

The lockdown affected my mental health more than anything, knowing that all the plans I had for when baby arrived can no longer be carried out, my parents still haven't met their granddaughter, it's difficult. Going into labour during the lockdown was quite difficult too, we had to have my Sister- in-Law isolate with us so that I would have a lift to the hospital, due to my partner only having a motorbike. As I said before even now that Baby is here we still can't do all the things we would normally do with a newborn, we can't have a newborn photo shoot, I wasn't able to have bounty pictures in the hospital. Although I cannot thank the Midwives in Glangwili Hospital enough, it was difficult not being able to have my partner with me on the ward and not able to have any visitors. I felt very lonely and isolated knowing that my partner was at home and I was in the hospital without anyone to talk to.

The Midwives on ward and Health Care Assistants were absolutely amazing, very helpful and will go the extra mile for all the patients.

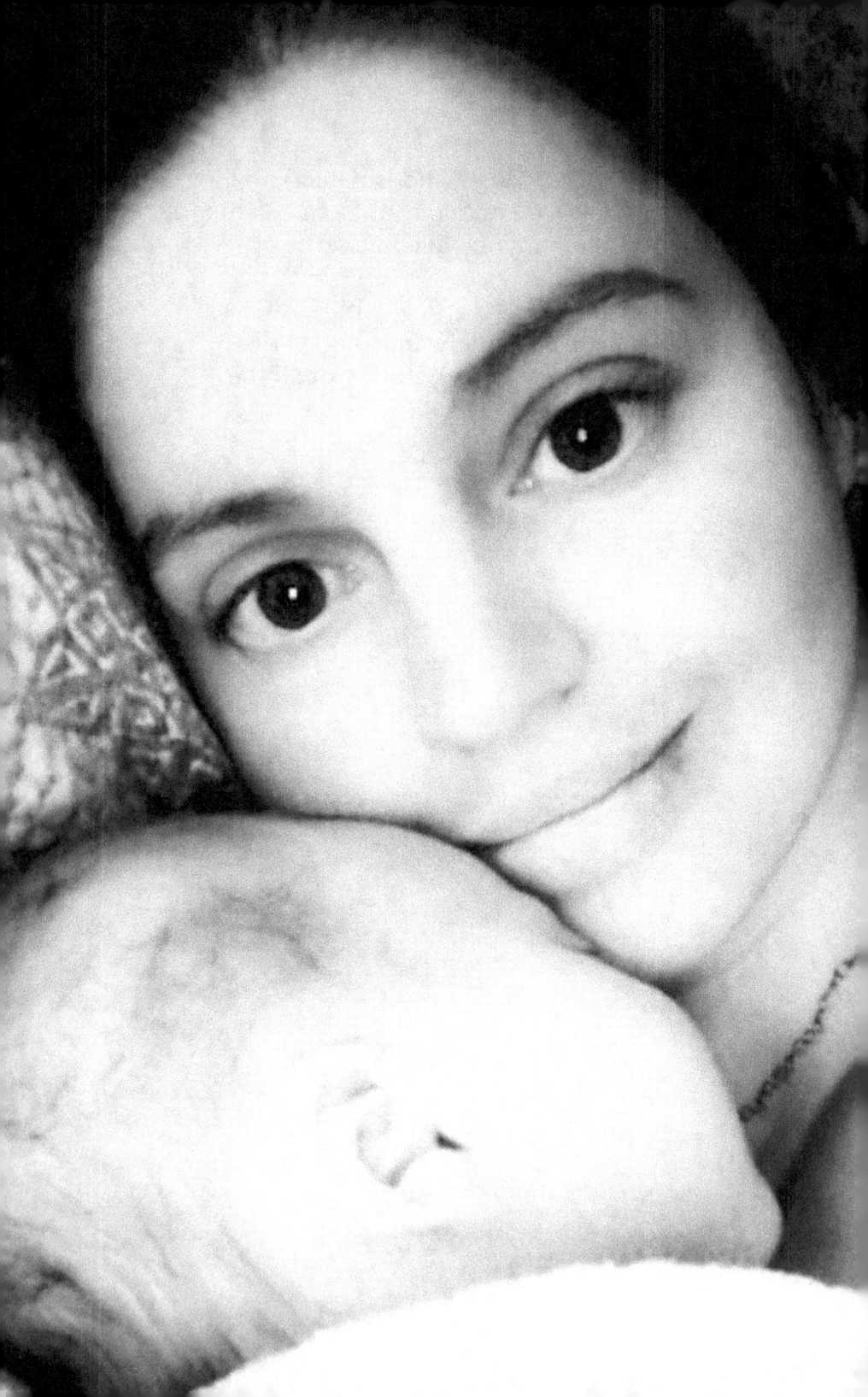

No. 9

Kimberly's Story

I would just like to say after all the stresses of pregnancy and everything that's going on with covid-19 at the moment I was very worried about giving birth. However, my little man arrived at home in the pool just as I wanted. My Midwife couldn't of done a better job of keeping me relaxed throughout the whole thing, Sorry for not giving you time to get all the bits ready, or waiting for the second Midwife to arrive but at least he wasn't as quick as my last one when the Midwife had a surprise in the ambulance. I really had no need to be worried as my Midwife was fantastic and giving birth at home was a very relaxing experience.

The covid-19 totally changed my plans for labour, I was dreading the birth. All I have ever wanted was a water birth and on my previous two I wasn't allowed, one due to being induced and the second due to complications. So, once I heard we were no longer allowed waterbirths at Withybush Midwife Led Unit or Carmarthen Midwife Led Unit I was very upset. I had growth scans as I was Consultant led until 37 due to previous pregnancy complications. My partner took time off for all appointments, but he missed the final scan and the last two Consultant appointments due to the covid-19 procedures and not being allowed in with me. It affected my mental health as my last Midwife appointment at 36 weeks I took in no information and cried the whole time due to having to do it alone, I have no recollection of anything the Midwife asked at the appointment and all I wanted to do was leave.

I opted for a home birth after hearing that although it wasn't advised I could have a water birth at home if that's what I wanted, So after speaking to my Midwife I chose to give birth at home.

I had alternate plans put into place in the event a Midwife couldn't come to my home, after my last experience I was dreading giving birth again.

I couldn't have my mum there for support during the birth due to restrictions on only having one person. I also couldn't have the photographer present to record the birth either. Everything I had envisioned was taken away due to covid-19.

Postnatally, I am five days postnatal and no one except my Midwife and my children have seen our son. My stepchildren have also been affected as they have yet to meet him and we have no idea how long it will be before they get to meet their little brother and have their first cuddle, None of my friends or family have met or cuddled him and it's like a repeat of my last pregnancy where no one was allowed to touch my daughter. His birth hasn't really been celebrated as I've not seen anyone to celebrate, My baby shower was also cancelled, so all the presents my friends and family got for him will have to wait till after lockdown in order to receive them.

The one positive to covid-19, is that we had time to bond as a family and it's been nice to not have to worry about people visiting and being able to just relax and enjoy our first few days.

So everything changed, three months ago I would have said you were mad if you told me I was going to give birth at home in my pool without any pain relief and just with my partner and a Midwife.

However, the experience in itself was beautiful, calm and serene. Being at home I had all my home comforts, and two hours after giving birth I was cuddled up in my own bed looking at my miracle, The support from the Midwife couldn't of been better and she kept me relaxed throughout the entire experience.

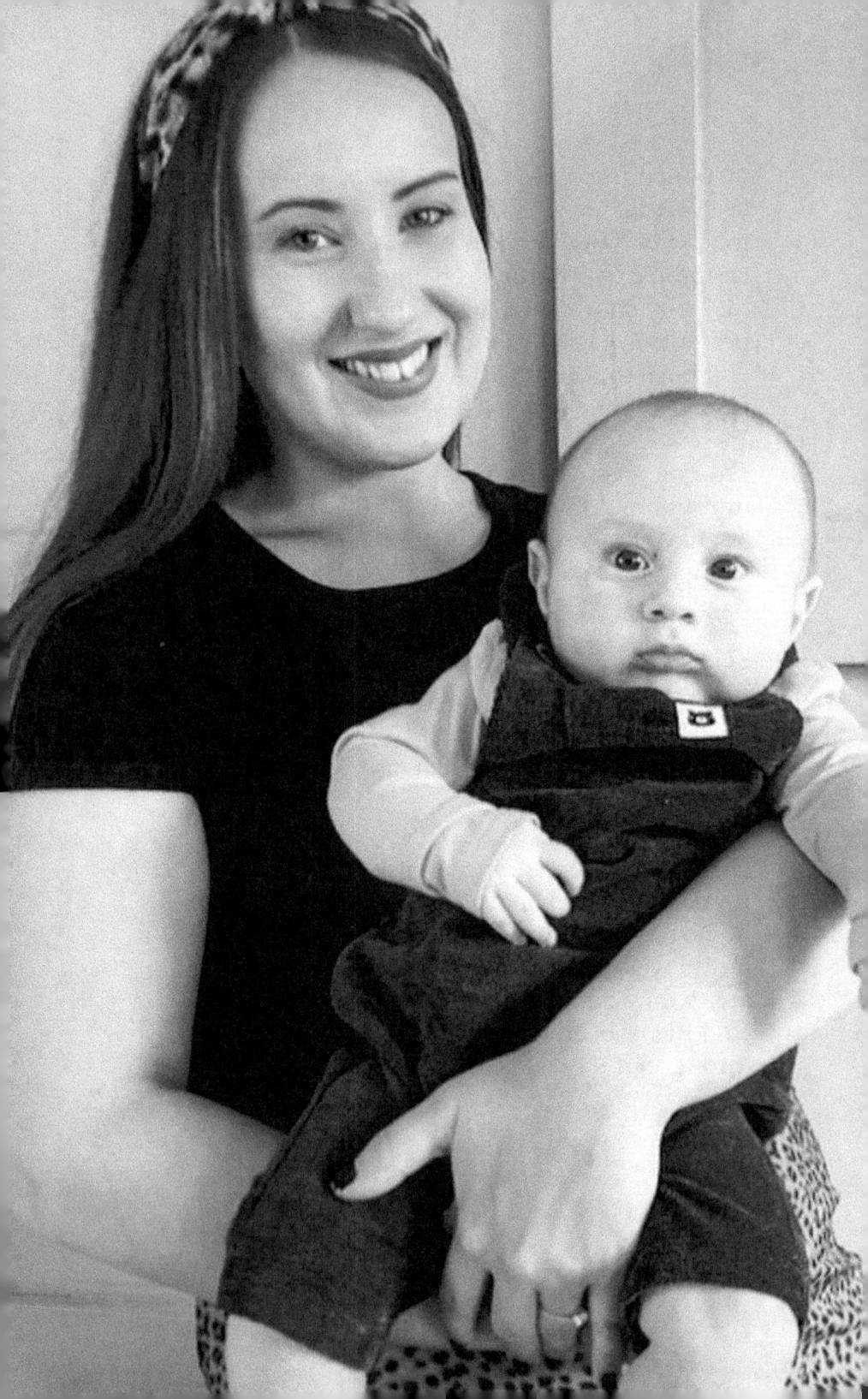

No. 10
Becky's Story

Such a strange and surreal time. It's definitely a story to tell my children when they are older. So here is my story. I was one of many women that gave birth in a global pandemic. So Back in July 2019, I found out I was five weeks pregnant. I felt excited, overwhelmed and anxious all a mixture of emotions. Earlier on in the year at the end of March I fell pregnant but unfortunately it didn't work out and I had a miscarriage at six weeks. So as time went on, I felt I was so lucky to fall pregnant again. But we kept it on the low down until my twelve weeks scan.

Weeks went by, we couldn't wait to find out the gender of our baby. We had a gender reveal party which was lovely. So special to celebrate with all our family and friends, the sex of our Baby. We found out were expecting a Baby boy.

It's now the beginning of 2020, it's the first time we hear about the coronavirus on the news. I remember watching the news and thinking to myself it's so sad what these people are going through in China and Italy. I never imagined it would ever reach us here. I had a notification on my phone "breaking news" first case of coronavirus in England. That's when it started to sink in, that this is real life and this virus is getting closer and it is really serious.

I tried to keep calm and not get myself too anxious or worried. When it came out on the news couple of months later that pregnant women are at high risk and they need to be isolated for three months. That is when reality hit me. I had been isolating for three weeks but I had to leave the house one day to go to my Midwife appointment. I remember my journey to the cottage hospital where I have my Midwife appointments, feeling anxious about leaving the house. I felt paranoid as soon as I left the car if I touch anything, constantly sterilizing my hands. My Fiancé waited in the car for me while I went into my appointment. I was gutted for him that he couldn't share this moment with me, like listening to our Baby heartbeat.

My midwife made me feel very comfortable. Any questions I had, she reassured me at all times. She explained that once I reached active labour, my fiancé could be there with me for the birth of our son. I totally understood but I couldn't help feeling upset, scared and worried. I was devastated when I found out only one birthing partner, I would have loved to have had my mum there for the birth. I had Tears rolling down my face knowing that I couldn't have my mum there holding my hand for the birth. Also, my fiancé had to wait in the car until I was in active labour. Not having that proud moment of all my family and friends to meet our baby boy for the first time. Not able to have visitors into the hospital. Most importantly not seeing my fiancé while we stayed in hospital for a couple of days after the birth. Everything felt so unnatural emotions were high.

The day finally came and it's the 7th April I'm 39 weeks pregnant approximately 8.00am I've woken up feeling abit under the weather. I was having mini contractions every few minutes. Very light but bearable. I thought I would get myself ready for the day, but the pains started to get worse, so I decided to ring my Community Midwife for some advice. I spoke to my Midwife on the phone and she's was very helpful, she advises me to ring antenatal and go from there. Due to a few complications through my pregnancy due to Group B Strep they advise me to come up to the ward for a monitoring. It's now 12pm we take a trip to the hospital. This moment in time I feel anxious I walk into the hospital it's all seems so quiet. Very surreal not a person around I anxiously walking into antenatal and I was greeted by a few lovely midwives who made me feel at ease straight away. They took me to comfortable area where it was spotless. Time passed but I wasn't in established labour and my Midwife was happy for me to go home. It looked like I was in very early stages of labour but nothing happening yet.

Hours went by and my contractions seemed to get worse. It's now 10 pm I am in a lot of discomfort, I feel anxious, scared about all the uncertainty in this world I knew my baby was coming very soon and it was such a bittersweet feeling. I was so excited to bring my son into the world, but never imagine I would bring him into a world with all this going on.

As I got to the hospital finally it was around 22.40. I walked through the main entrance doors my eyes filling up with tears. I was exhausted and in extreme pain, I don't know how I did it. I managed to power walk into the Antenatal ward Where I had two lovely Midwives waiting there for me. I felt relief that I was there, and I felt safe. It was quiet, not another patient around, I walked into the ward and my lovely Midwife made me feel very comfortable. From that very moment, I felt okay.

The Midwife explained to me that she was going to get the drip to be prepared ready for birth. As she left my waters had broken all over the floor, I manage to get myself on to the bed ring the buzzer. The Midwife came in to examine me and she said I was 8cm dilated so I quickly grab my phone and text my fiancé to come meet me. As he had to wait in the car until I was ready to give birth. Within five minutes of him walking into the room I was in I had given birth to our beautiful baby boy. So, it was only 10 minutes from walking into the hospital and my waters had broken and I had given birth. The most craziness surreal moment in my life. It was the quickest birth ever; it was all done in a matter of five minutes. Luckily, my partner was with me he just made the birth. I had to stay in hospital for two nights. My partner Adam was able to stay with me for a little while after birth to enjoy this moment just the three of us. He dressed our little boy gave him his first bottle; they were precious moments.

Later that evening, I was taking in a wheelchair up to Dinefwr ward. my Midwife took me to my bed, and I felt very comfortable and at ease. I had to say goodbye to my fiancé as I knew I wouldn't see him for two days as there was no visitors on the ward. I could not of ask for better Midwife who looked after my baby and myself. It all felt so natural like nothing was going on in this world. Yes, they were wearing gowns, gloves and they even had masks on, but I respected that for all of our safety. The days went by, and everything was so professional and relaxed. I didn't feel anxious at all, I knew we were in the right care. The ward was very clean, and you could tell that extra precautions had been put in place. They were consequently wiping surfaces and mopping floors.

I can't thank the Midwife's and Healthcare's, and Domestics enough. They always had a smile on their faces and time for me. We were in the best of hands I am so overwhelmed with the experience it was incredible, myself and my baby were in the best of care. Even though, it is only normal to feel upset and lonely not having my family around me when I needed them the most. I didn't feel like I was on my own, I was in the best of hands and I cannot thank them enough.

Two days later, and we are able to go home. I was exhausted, but so excited to be back in the comfort of my own home. The journey home seems so peaceful there was hardly any cars on the road. But the police had set up two roadblocks on the way back. It was daunting, but we fully understand why they are doing it for our own safety.

I finally arrived home and walked back into my house with my baby boy in my arms. My little girl was waiting for me to come home. We are safe and we are all content staying home seemed so easy. The four of us were so happy our family back together and everything felt so positive and there was all this sadness and negativity going on in the world but the one thing I'll never forget is this experience bringing my son into the world.

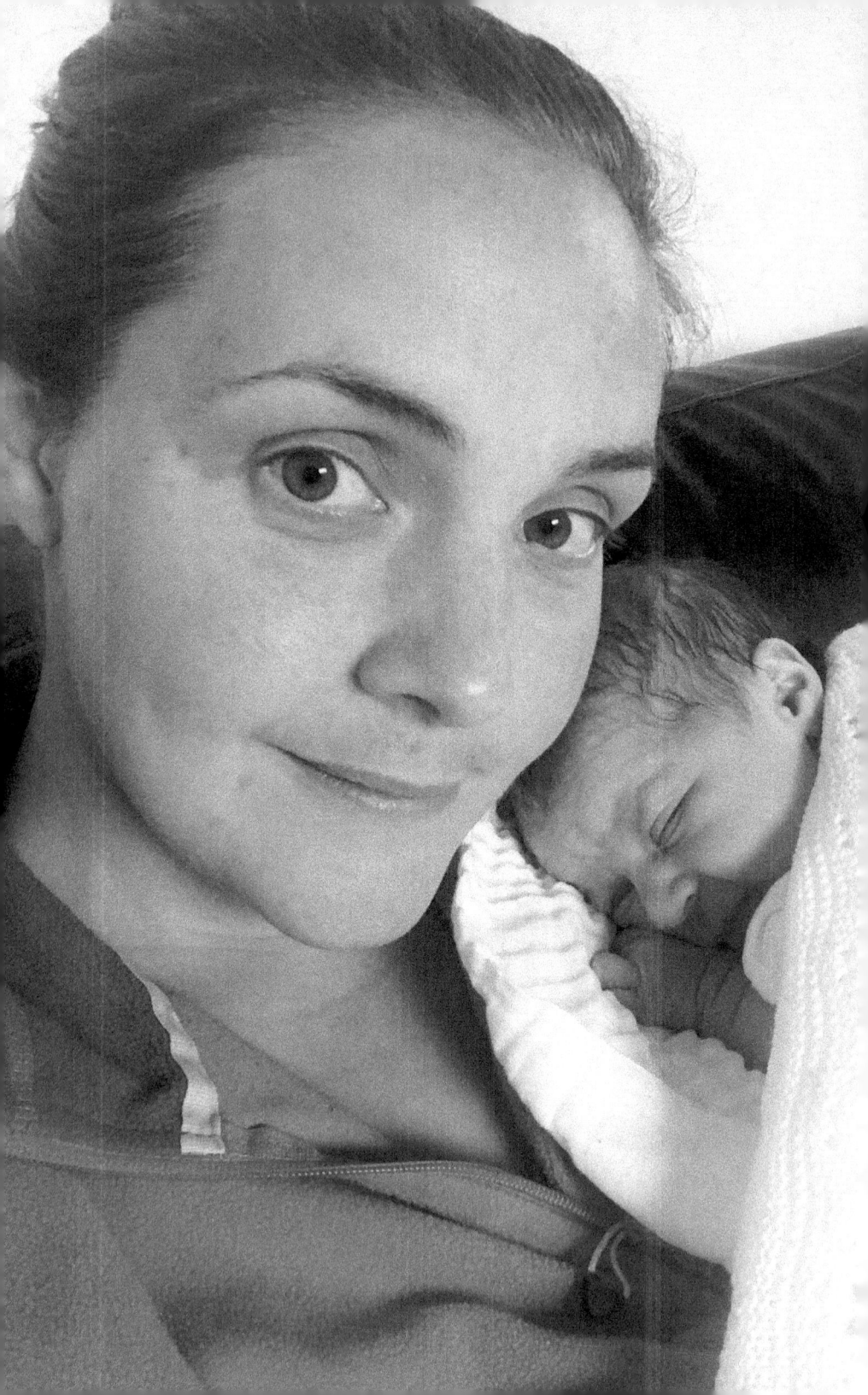

No. 11

Charlotte's Story

We first found out the wonderful news when I went for my three yearly smear test as the nurse suspected I might be pregnant and asked when I was due my next period. As it was due that week, I didn't think anything of it.

The following week we found out that we were expecting. We were elated, we knew we always wanted another but didn't expect it to happen as we had such trouble conceiving our first child. Thankfully, my partner was able to come with me to the twenty- week scan where we found out we were having another little girl. We were over the moon!

After hearing about the covid-19 I noticed things started to change. I was receiving letters to go to antenatal appointments, but they were different this time I was asked to attend on my own. I think if this would have been my first pregnancy it would have really affected me, but I took it all in my stride and just went with it. On the next scan the baby started to measure small and I wish I had someone there for moral support. I didn't know how to feel about it, and I felt like I had nobody to talk to.

As baby was measuring small, I was having to go for growth scans every two weeks to check her growth. This really made me anxious as I knew then that I would have to visit the hospital more frequently and I would have to go to all the appointments on my own. Every time I went to the hospital I noticed small changes were being made, sanitisers used more frequently, signs up everywhere saying to use them, wash your hands for up to 20 seconds, please don't attend clinics if you have a cough or temperature etc.

Then on the last few appointments there was tape placed across seats to ensure people were sitting the correct distance apart, Midwives/Nurses wearing face masks and disposable aprons. During my last appointment at 37 weeks where I was told that baby was growing and there was nothing to worry about, I was told that they were no longer doing water births at the hospital. I was devastated, I didn't think I could do it without the water as it helped take away the pain last time. I really hoped it would change and prayed that I would go over my due date as things might change in time, but they didn't.

The day finally came where I started to feel contractions. I wanted to stay at home as long as I could as I knew that my partner wasn't allowed to come in until I was in established labour. The contractions started coming every ten minutes and then I started panicking thinking that this was happening, and I would have been on my own in the hospital. I was so scared!! By the time we got to the hospital my contractions were coming every four minutes. My partner took me to the ward door and then had to leave me until I had been checked over. It was 21:30 at this point. The Midwives were amazing and put me at ease straightaway. I was examined and told the fantastic news that I was in established labour and that my partner could be phoned. I was elated!!

After what seemed like twenty minutes on my own (it was probably only five minutes) he arrived, and everything started to happen. The Midwives wore all the protective gear, but not once did I think or start to worry about the covid-19, I just wanted my baby out safely. Contractions started coming quickly and by 23:45 baby Cerys was born. The care we received was outstanding, not once did we feel on our own, at risk or the baby would be at risk. The ladies did their job and still mopped my brow to helpcool me down in labour. They were amazing.

Since being home it has been a little different, no actual visitors, just lots of FaceTime with family and friends and a few came to the window to see the baby. I think our family have found it harder than we have as we have our own little unit in the house, and we have the unlimited cuddles with the baby. I do miss the fact that I know that I won't be able to go to baby groups this time, but a positive in all of this is I've managed to continue breast feeding longer than I had previously (I was really conscious before about doing it in public). It has only been six day's since she has been with us, but I know that we have a long way to go until this lockdown and covid-19 are behind us. But I would rather be away for my family for this short time and see them again than not at all.

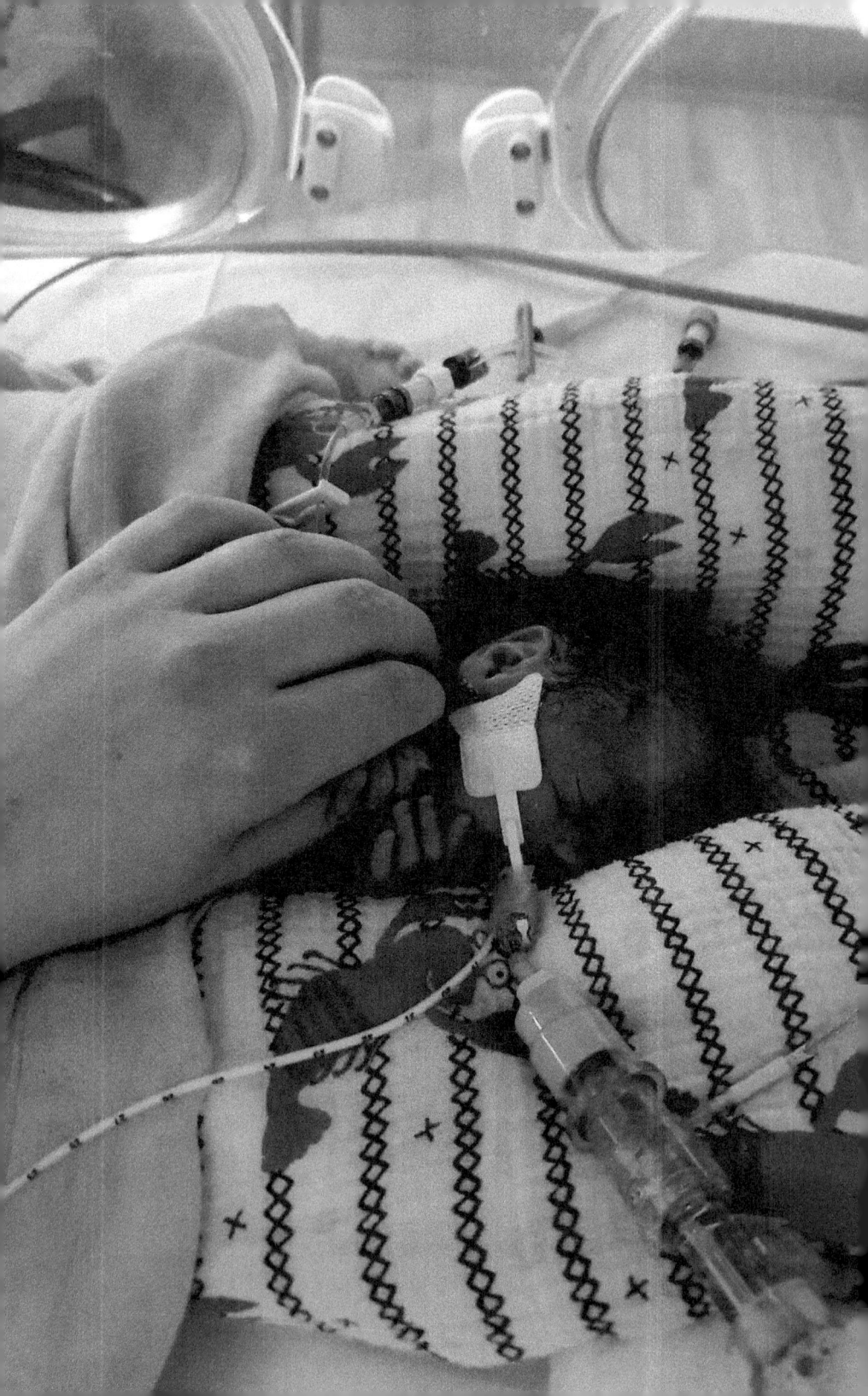

No. 12
Melissa's Story

Finding out I was pregnant with our fifth baby was a shock, and one of the first things to come to mind was what if we have another premature baby. So as soon as I could, I got booked under a Consultant who arranged to see me two weekly along with scans to check the baby and the cervix, we found out baby number five was our second boy! The cervical scans showed no reason that I would have another premature baby, I did have a chest infection around twenty weeks which was discussed as possible covid-19, but which was then proved to be a bad chest infection!

Around this time, I also experienced three very large gushes of water, but the hospital scanned and said it can't have been waters as your little boy has plenty around him, so it was left as that. Then on Thursday 9th April I woke up to a lot of blood, clots and a toilet full of blood as well as pressure pains so was admitted to hospital who gave me two doses of steroids to help babies lungs should he be born prematurely, as well as the sliding scale to help with diabetes. After two days in the hospital I was still bleeding so it was decided I'd be kept in another 24 hours and the same again the following day!

On the Sunday I felt very off but all my observations were fine so it was put down to a possible side effect from the steroids but then at 1pm I felt a trickle after a wee, then another, so I laid on the bed for fifteen minutes then sat up to a gush. I knew straight away it was my waters, so the midwife checked for me and it was premature rupture of membranes again at just 25 weeks! Shortly after I was taken to the labour ward just in case, as I previously had fast labours with my girls. As my temperature was 37.9, I had to go into a room for suspected covid-19! I had to wear a face mask, anything I touched had to be binned and very minimal staff footfall into the room, I was given magnesium sulphate for the baby's brain protection. While there it was picked up that the baby was having bradycardia and tachycardia episodes, so they started to prepare me for a category 1 caesarean section! I was on my own and petrified of being put to sleep! But then his heart rate suddenly settled so they decided to hang fire...

His heart rate continued to be ok but then my temperature started to creep up, 38, 38.5, 39, where it peaked at just short of 40.2oc! For me, my normal is 36.6, my heart rate had shot up to the 200s and I was delirious at this stage. It was decided that I needed to be moved to a hospital that had an intensive care bed for me! I asked about the Baby when they considered a local hospital and the reply I got was that his prognosis isn't good, I found a little energy in me to go with the transfer and it was decided I go to another hospital in Wales which have Neonatal facilities for the baby.

An ambulance came to take me and I had a million people talking to me , trying to get blood, and trying to insert cannulas. They put me on oxygen (under my mask) and put me in the back of the ambulance, the ride actually did me good as they had the windows open and it cooled me down!

When I arrived in the next hospital, I was taken to a big empty bay where everyone was gowned up and swabbed me for Covid 19! I had Neonatal and Obstetric Doctor's come in and speak to me, again giving a poor prognosis based on how poorly I was, they gave me an option of having a caesarean section which he may not survive and I may have to be put to sleep for or induction of labour. I chose induction and was given twelve hours to get him out, I had the hormone drip as well as a massive cocktail of other drugs including antibiotics which helped to stabilise me. I was checked for dilation and no change, so the drip was turned up.

I was checked again there was no change, so the drip was turned up again to 24, still no contractions! At this point my Covid swab came back! Negative! So, I was able to take off the mask, breathe properly and go to the labour ward!

They gave me the option try a higher dose of the drip but risk potential scar rupture or a caesarean section, as the scar rupture risk was still small we tried to increase it up to 36...they checked again still no dilation, he said he never turns it up this high in women who have had previous caesarean sections but turned it up again to 48! A few small niggles but an hour later no change! So, at this stage a caesarean section was the only option left.

Consent forms were signed and I was taken to theatre, as my bump was so small they said they may have to cut upwards instead of across to get to him, also there was a high risk of hysterectomy and bleeding, I said just do what you can to get him out safely, I don't care what my body looks like and I although a hysterectomy would be a big thing I wouldn't need it for any more babies. They started the surgery and I couldn't stop shaking through the medications and I guess fear, then we heard a little cry(the baby had been born)and he was okay!

The Neonatal team set to work and ventilated him straight away, I got to see him before they took him to Neonatal intensive care unit and Daddy got a photo something that didn't happen with Xavier and I was extremely grateful for! He weighed 1lb 11oz exactly 1lb lighter than Xavier. So now we are on our journey with Theodore, an unexpected second Neonatal intensive care journey. It was only after he was born it was confirmed I had in fact had sepsis, a severe Staphylococcal infection and after his birth I was on intravenous antibiotics. Once it was confirmed what infection it was decided that I go on intra venous antibiotics for two weeks, four times a day!

So that is our story now as I write the rest of it continues, at the moment Theodore is smashing Neonatal intensive care and showing who is boss, and we hope this is how he will continue!

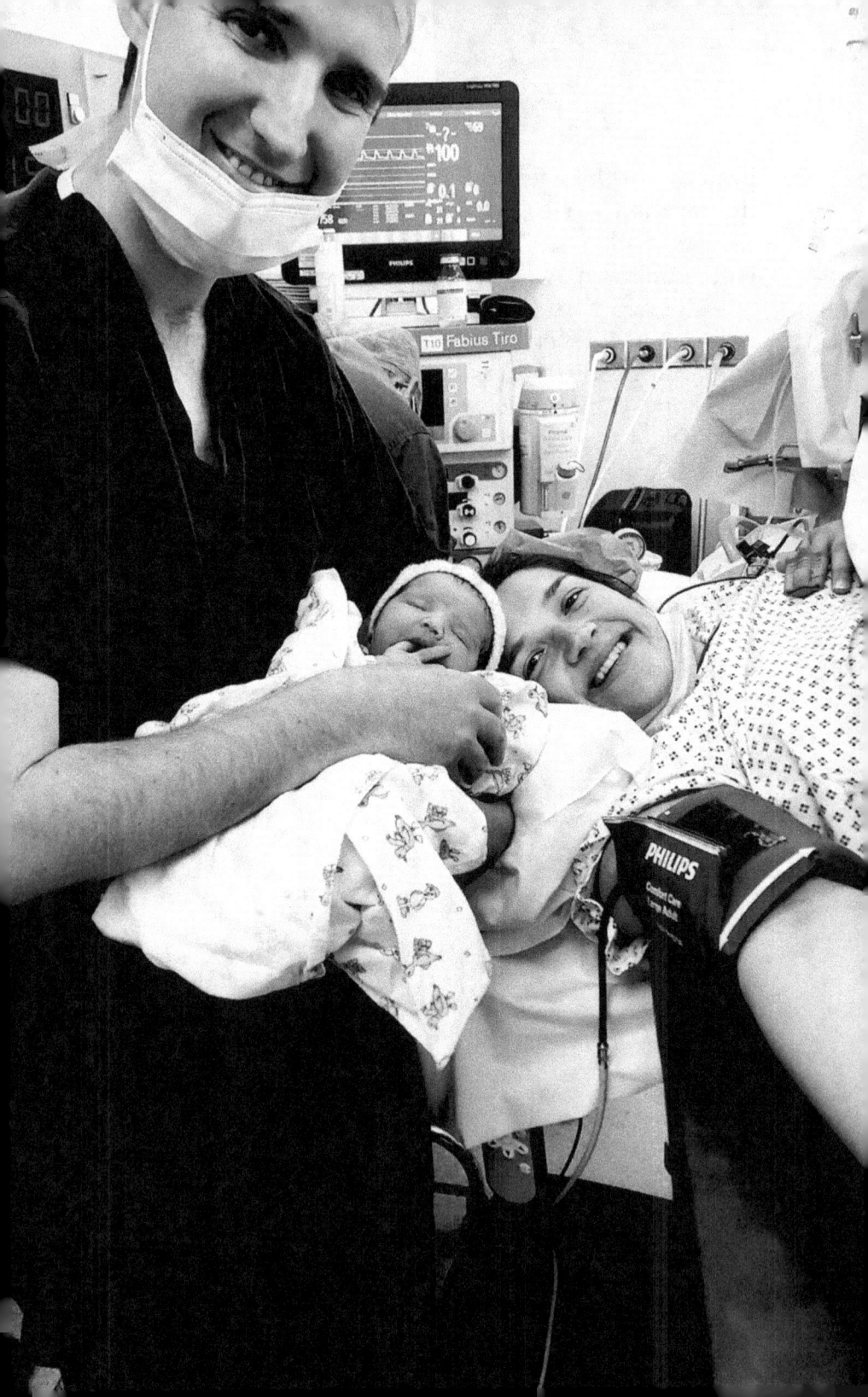

No. 13

Holly's Story

When I first found out about coronavirus, I remember how devastating and rapid the spread had been in China and convinced it wouldn't reach the UK.

It wasn't until a week before lockdown that I realised the seriousness when the news showed hospitalisation numbers were increasing by the day and people were bulk buying, and I was stood behind a fully grown man crying in Boots whose wife had just a baby, and he was struggling and panicking to buy baby formula, that was when I realised the effect this virus was going to have.

I usually took my toddler to my antenatal appointments but now a big sign had been put up saying no children, and the waiting room was full of pregnant women sat in silence and spaced two metres apart with all the staff in full protective clothing and masks, it was a very different experience.

I was always due to have an elective caesarean section due to a third-degree tear with my first, but I was very concerned it would be cancelled or I would have to go alone.

Mine and my partners family all live in

Monmouthshire and both sets of parents are shielding and couldn't cross the border due to the restrictions, so we had to rely on friends to have our three year old, to be able to go for the caesarean-section. This was devastating as none of our family could come and support us.

I can honestly say I had a really supportive experience last Wednesday having an elective caesarean-section to give birth to my daughter Primrose.

From the beginning my partner stayed with me until we went down to theatre and the whole team were really great the Midwives, Health Care Assistant's, Anaesthetic and Obstetric team of Doctors, Nurses and ODP's, were fab and friendly. They all introduced themselves and were really friendly and told me exactly what was happening throughout!

It didn't go exactly to plan but I felt supported and happy throughout and my partner got to spend lovely time with our baby post caesarean-section whilst I recovered which was great.

Once back on the ward the Midwives and Health Care Assistants were really, really helpful and helped me care for my baby whilst I recovered and I was able to go home the next day and my partner met me and my baby girl at the ward. The ward is really peaceful which is the plus side of no visitors and focused on mums and babies!

My postnatal care has also been different as some appointments have been over the phone and we haven't been able to do have the traditional "red book" or get excited about registering her birth.

Our families are gutted they have had to meet their grandchild via FaceTime and not been able to have a cuddle or even stand outside the window as our toddler wouldn't understand why her grandparents can't come in or even touch her. They wait in anticipation for lockdown to be lifted as do we.

Our friends have been really great ranging from child care during birth (my friend self-isolated for two weeks to have my toddler) to even sending hampers to help my partner who is also single handed doing home schooling, supporting me post caesarean and running around after a newborn.

Lockdown has given my family time to adjust from a three to a four and this has been precious uninterrupted time. It has also allowed my partner extended paternity to bond with our daughter Primrose and help the bond with her sister Penelope that has been able to flourish.

All I can say is thank you as I was dreading it, and was very anxious about having my baby in lockdown and my partner not spending time with our baby, he came in the ward with me to wait for the procedure and was allowed to stay until I was stable afterwards and it felt like a normal delivery! I can't thank all the team at Glangwili Hospital enough!

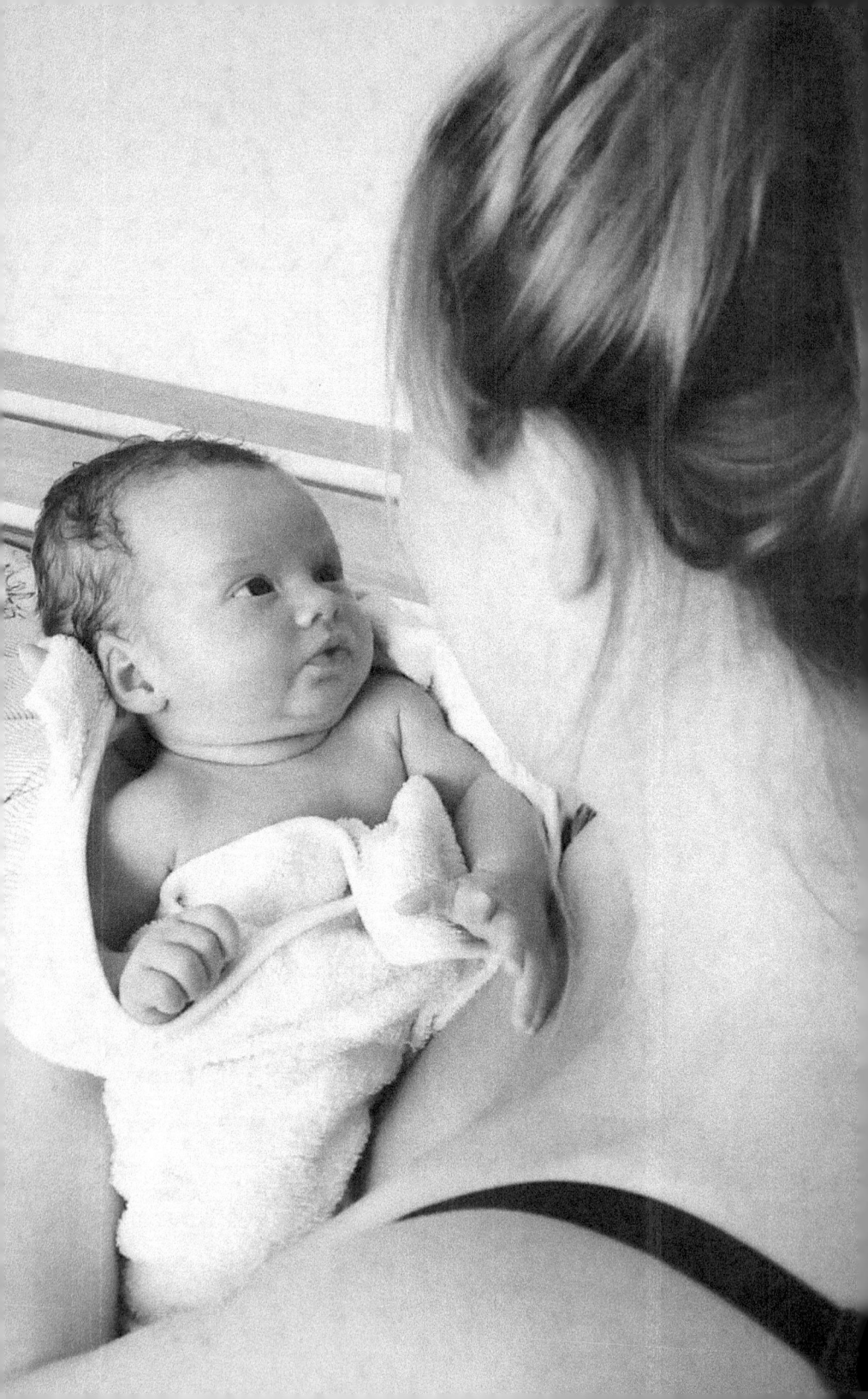

No. 14

Siana's Story

I am a first-time mum and had planned to give birth in the Midwife Led Unit at Glangwili Hospital as I wanted a natural delivery using a birth pool. With three weeks until my due date I found out that the Midwife Led Unit needed to be used for women with coronavirus to give birth and I was told I would have to deliver on the labour ward due to my baby having a dilated kidney. I wasn't happy with the idea, as I wanted to avoid any interventions and I was becoming more concerned about the risk of catching coronavirus if I had to stay in hospital. I also wanted my husband to be with me during and after labour. I spoke to my community Midwife and we changed my birth plan to having a homebirth instead.

My Midwife was really supportive, and I felt much more confident having taken back control over how I wanted my birth experience to be. I was worried that staff shortages due to coronavirus might mean that there wouldn't be Midwives available to attend my home for the birth, but luckily that wasn't a problem.

My labour started at 4am with regular mild contractions. Midwives came to examine me at 11am and confirmed I was in the early stages of labour. They had to wear full PPE but reassured me they were the same lovely caring people under the face masks! They really put me at ease.

At 4pm a midwife returned to our house and confirmed I was in active labour. For the next few hours, I laboured using a tens machine and then birth pool and gas and air for pain relief.

At 9pm my waters were artificially broken to speed up the labour. This worked well but unfortunately as I approached transition at around midnight our Midwife had to swap as she had already had a very long shift.

As the new Midwives took over, I began to feel the urge to push but unfortunately my baby's heart rate dropped, and the midwives decided that I should be transferred to hospital. We live an hour's drive from Glangwili Hospital but luckily baby's heart rate stabilised in the ambulance and he was born halfway to the hospital at the side of the road!

Even though our birth didn't go exactly according to plan, I am still really happy with the choices we made and the care we received from the Community Midwives who supported my birth choices and made us feel safe and comfortable in a really difficult time. We are now settled into life with our gorgeous little boy who is now three weeks old and we are loving every moment!

We are loving being new parents, I think without the pressure/distraction of visitors we have had such a peaceful relaxing time bonding.

Before our baby was born, I was worried that coronavirus might be more harmful to pregnant women than the general public (although now it looks like that's not the case). Because of this I started my maternity leave earlier than I had planned so that I could fully isolate at home before the lockdown was imposed.

My appointments with the Midwife and all scans went ahead as planned, but for my final few appointments with the Midwife she had to wear PPE and brought me into the health centre through a side entrance to avoid people in the waiting area.

The biggest impact that the virus has had on us, is that my mum wasn't able to be my second birth partner, and none of our family have been able to meet our baby yet. As my mum was not allowed with us for the birth, we had her on video call for the whole thing. My dad and sister ended up joining the video call too which was actually really amazing, I had everyone there supporting me! We are just hoping our family can meet our baby soon, my mum has really struggled not being allowed to hold her first grandchild. We are feeling quite anxious about the idea of life after lockdown and letting people have cuddles with the worry of infection.

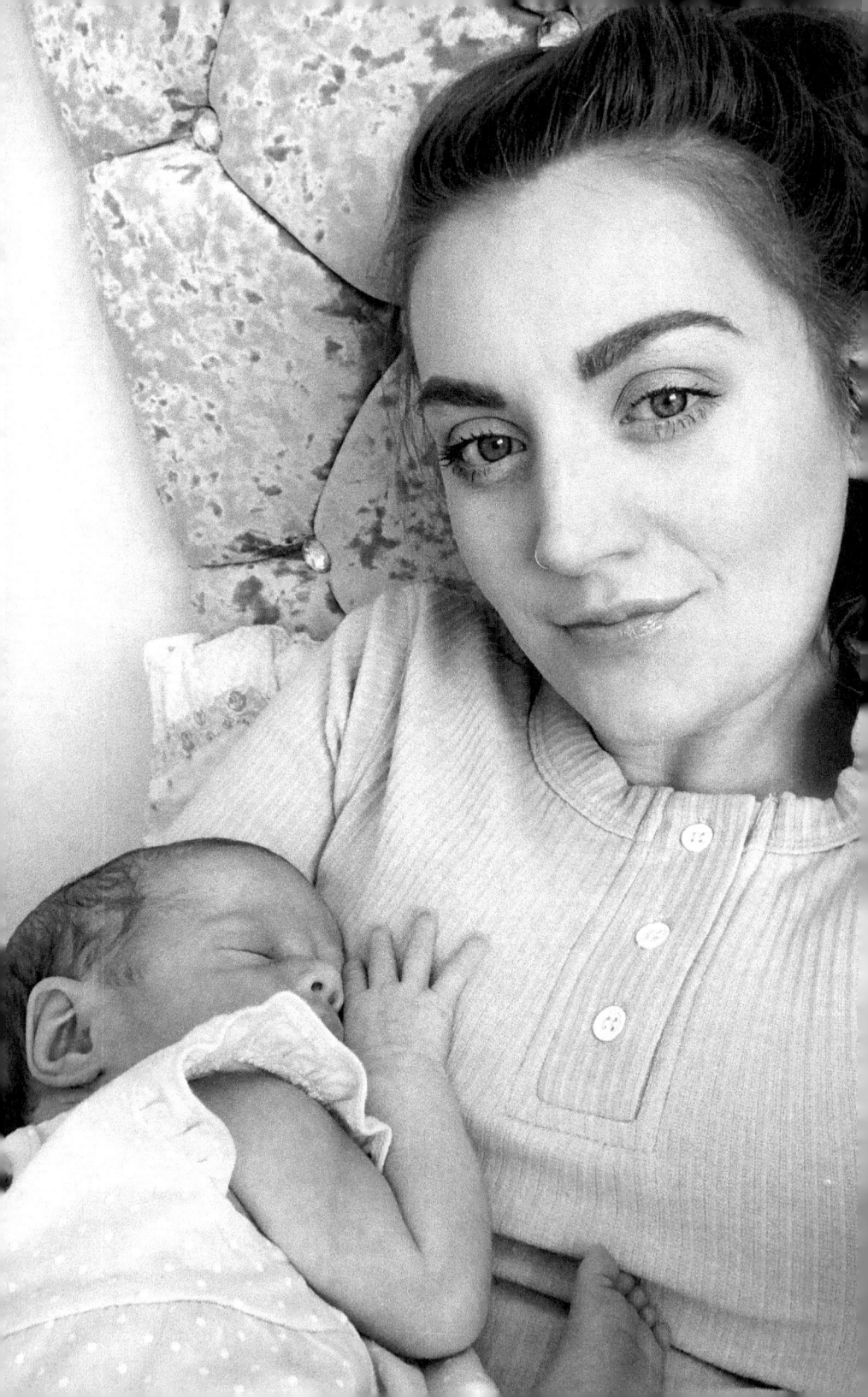

No. 15

Chelsea's Story

Obviously at first, we didn't really think anything of the coronavirus and thought it would only affect other countries, little did we know it would soon end up coming to Wales. I think after my baby shower, which was on March 15th, we started to realise how serious the coronavirus was. After this I ended up self-isolating to protect me and my unborn baby. This was a difficult time as I was at home on my own as my partner still had to go to work, with over a month still to go until I was due to give birth we didn't know what to expect.

As time went on and the country was told we had to go into lockdown anxiety struck and I started getting scared as to what would happen regarding the birth of my little baby girl.

As my baby was breech from week 31, appointments carried on as usual and went from every two weeks to weekly appointments to make sure baby was safe. I had regular scans to keep an eye on baby's position, but she was too comfortable and at week 36 we decided as she still hadn't moved that a caesarean-section would be the best option. My partner was unable to attend the scans in the last few weeks which I found hard as I felt quite alone. Midwives appointments in the surgery carried on, we had to sit outside in the car until the midwife was ready to see me & would call me in. Everything felt very confusing and I did not expect the end of my pregnancy to happen that way.

When I went in for my scan appointments, all the woman had to sit two meters apart. Scary times!

The decided the caesarean-section was planned for 39+6 weeks, so as planned me and my partner turned up at the hospital where we were greeted by the Midwives on duty. Considering everything that was going on, I felt calm and relaxed regardless. Everything went well with the section and my beautiful baby girl was born 22nd April 11.31am.

After being out of theatre for an hour, my partner was made to leave as there was no visitors allowed on the ward, as I had an epidural I was very tired and sleepy so didn't really mind that he had to leave. As soon as the medication wore off and I realised I was on my own then I started feeling emotional. Thankfully, the nurses and midwives on duty that night/day were amazing and couldn't do enough to help as I couldn't do much due to having the caesarean-section.

The next day I was told I would be able to leave at lunchtime which I couldn't wait for as it meant I got to go home and spend the night at home with my new family. It was very strange leaving as the midwife had to wheel me to the main entrance of the hospital as my partner could not come up to the ward.

The only thing that has been heartbreaking during this time is that our families have not been able to meet her yet. This being my father's first grandchild he has been absolutely devastated in not being able to have a cuddle with his first little grandchild.

At the moment it is almost time for my partner to go back to work and I'm finding that very difficult.

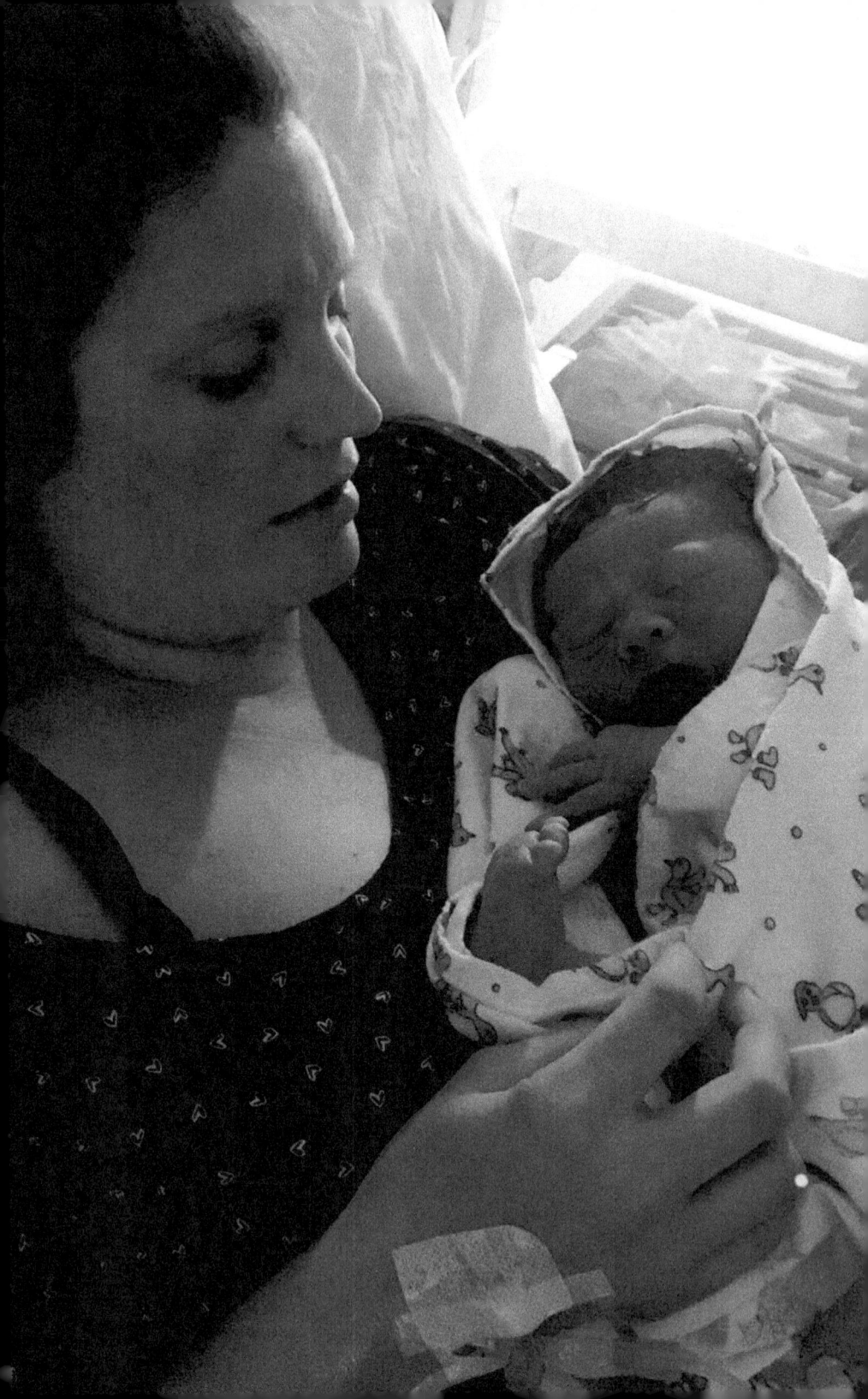

No. 16
Jennifer's Story

My pregnancy was an anxious time at the start. I have Hashimoto's disease and was under Consultant led care. I was at a high risk of miscarriage during the first trimester, I already have four children, all-natural births (aged 17, 14, 6 and 5) and have had four miscarriages. I had regular scans and saw my Consultant regularly, I started to feel less anxious by 21 weeks after my sixth scan, as baby was healthy and growing as he should. I was booked in for regular growth scans. At 28 weeks I had a Glucose tolerance test, my dad and aunty are both Type 1Diabetics, so I always had the test. This time though, for the first time I was told I had Gestational Diabetes, so I was transferred to care in Glangwili Hospital instead. I met with the Diabetic Midwives who were amazing. I had planned a home birth as I'd had with my previous two but was told I it was too high risk. So, the Diabetic Midwife arranged a review with the Consultant Midwife, who agreed I have Midwife Led Care but go up to the Labour ward if I needed to.

Two weeks before I was due, I started having hypos, so I was booked in for an induction of labour on the 17th March, at 39weeks. I was told then that I would have to stay in for 24hrs for monitoring after the baby was born. I found out due to the Covid my children wouldn't be allowed to visit me and meet their baby brother so I decided I would be far more comfortable, and safe at home. But unfortunately, my waters went on the 15th March, but labour didn't start so I had to go ahead and go for the induction of labour. I didn't know what to expect with never having been induced, and with Covid in the hospital. But I needn't have worried about being at the hospital, I wouldn't have known the covid-19 situation was going on. I was put at ease by the Midwives who were lovely. My son was born at 1.57am on 18th March 2020 , the labour was a lot harder than my previous four, and he got stuck, when he was born he was unresponsive and not breathing so they whisked him away to give him some oxygen, he was finally okay, and we got to hold him. We had to stay in hospital for a couple of days due to Freddie having a couple of hypos and a high temperature. My husband was allowed to stay with me, from the start until we went down to the ward and came back the following two days.

Since coming home no one has met our baby boy apart from his siblings, we haven't been anywhere apart from local walks, and it's great getting lots of time with him and the rest of the children, however I feel like we have been forgotten slightly, like he doesn't exist. We haven't been able to register his birth, and although the Health visitor phoned and did an assessment over the phone when he was ten days old, she never came out to weigh him or see how we are getting on and we haven't heard from her since. He's eight weeks old and due his first vaccinations next week and I had to ring the surgery to see what I'm supposed to do as normally the Health visitor tells you.

It's not a complaint about the NHS, I actually feel really happy just feel slightly like we are forgotten and I know that my baby is feeding well (breastfed) and gaining weight, and everything is ok as he's not my first, but I feel sad for the people who are first time mum's needing that extra support and not being able to get it.

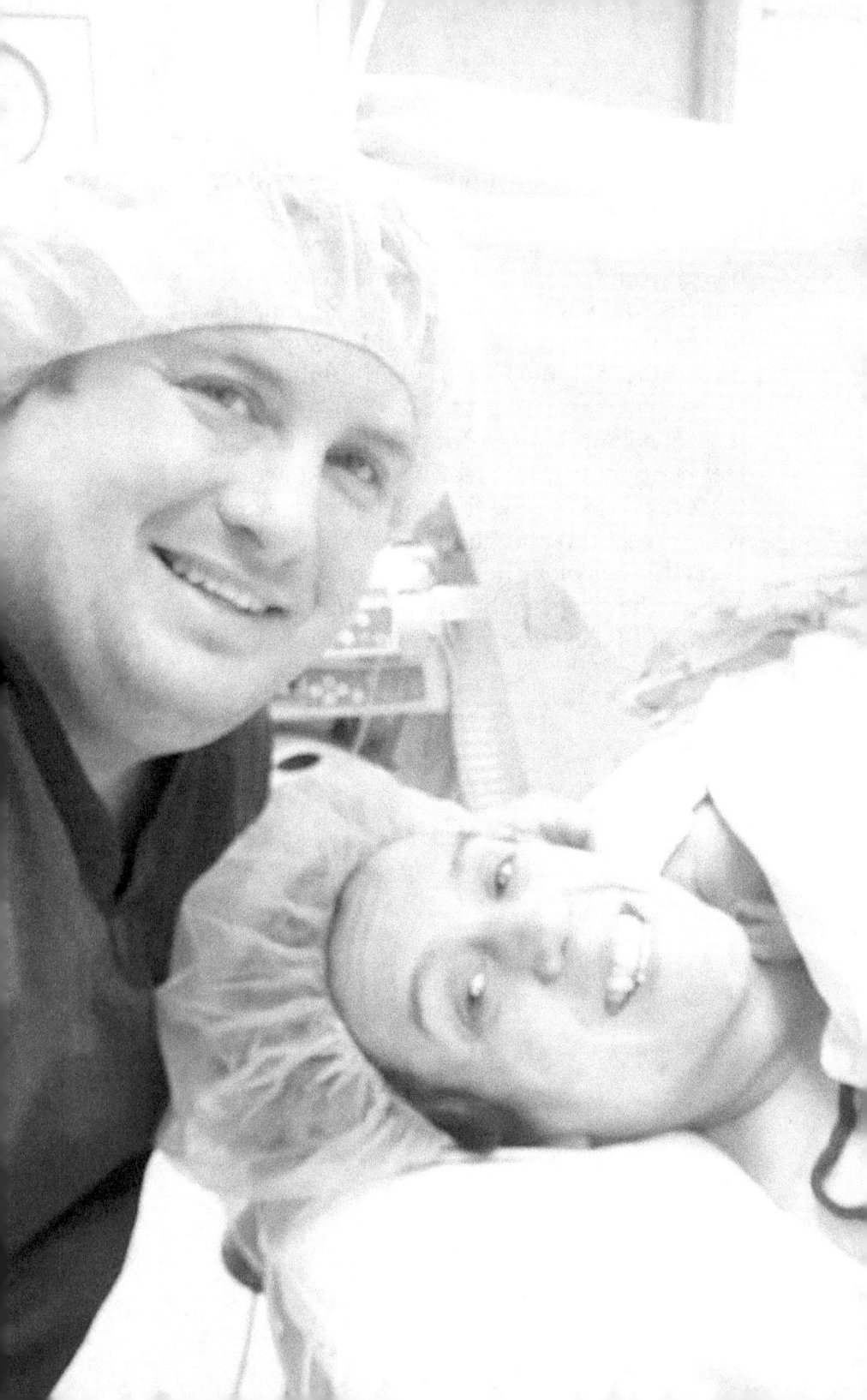

No. 17

Kate's Story

So, in the summer of 2019 I was delighted to find out I was pregnant with our second child. I was over the moon that my daughter would be a big sister. I was a little apprehensive due to a very worrying and challenging first pregnancy. (Which all turned out fine and I now have a chatty, busy 2-year-old). I knew I would be consultant led but had every confidence in the team at Withybush General Hospital as they had been so kind, caring and professional previously. My first and second trimester were really enjoyable, appointments came and went, and time went by so quickly. As I entered the third trimester covid 19 was beginning to become more of an issue though it still did not seem really to us in the UK.

I was really impressed with my care and felt that worries and thoughts were always put first. We had a really positive meeting with the Consultant midwife at Withybush Hospital and I felt confident going into the final weeks of my pregnancy. When it came to 36 weeks unfortunately covid-19 was very much with us which meant my husband could not attend antenatal appointments with me. However, the staff at Withybush Hospital were great and put my mind at ease. Being in the waiting room with women all in the same boat actually struck up conversation and allowed an opportunity to discuss worries and experiences, I do not think this would have happened had we all had partners there.

Due to a few minor complications at 38 weeks it was decided that my baby should be delivered by semi elective section. So, I was admitted as an inpatient to Glangwili Hospital on a Thursday afternoon. Again, with only partners permitted on the ward it allowed the women on the ward to chat and bond during this surreal time.

I cannot fault my care and support during my short stay in Glangwili Hospital. From my fantastic midwife to the whole team during the caesarean-section I felt safe and secure at all time. It was of course strange not having visitors to meet baby Betsi but if anything, it allowed precious bonding time for me and Stephen. I was out twenty-four hours after the caesarean section and felt ready to come home, this was my second caesarean section so I was probably a bit more prepared than I would have been. All of the staff from the Health care assistants to the Baby Doctors were supportive and caring at all times.

The hardest part of my whole birth experience were the weeks afterwards. Betsi is now seven weeks and still yet to meet grandparents, aunties and uncles, cousins and friends. I am home with a toddler and newborn for twelve-hour days alone. My husband is a farmer and it is his busiest season. So emotionally and socially this has been the polar opposite to what I experienced with my first. This is where I think covid-19 has affected me the most. My midwife and health visitor appointments were very strange and although they did their very best in this situation, I felt they were unable to give you the time they wanted to due to restrictions.

However, I now have two beautiful daughters, all thanks to the Hywel Dda University Health Board.

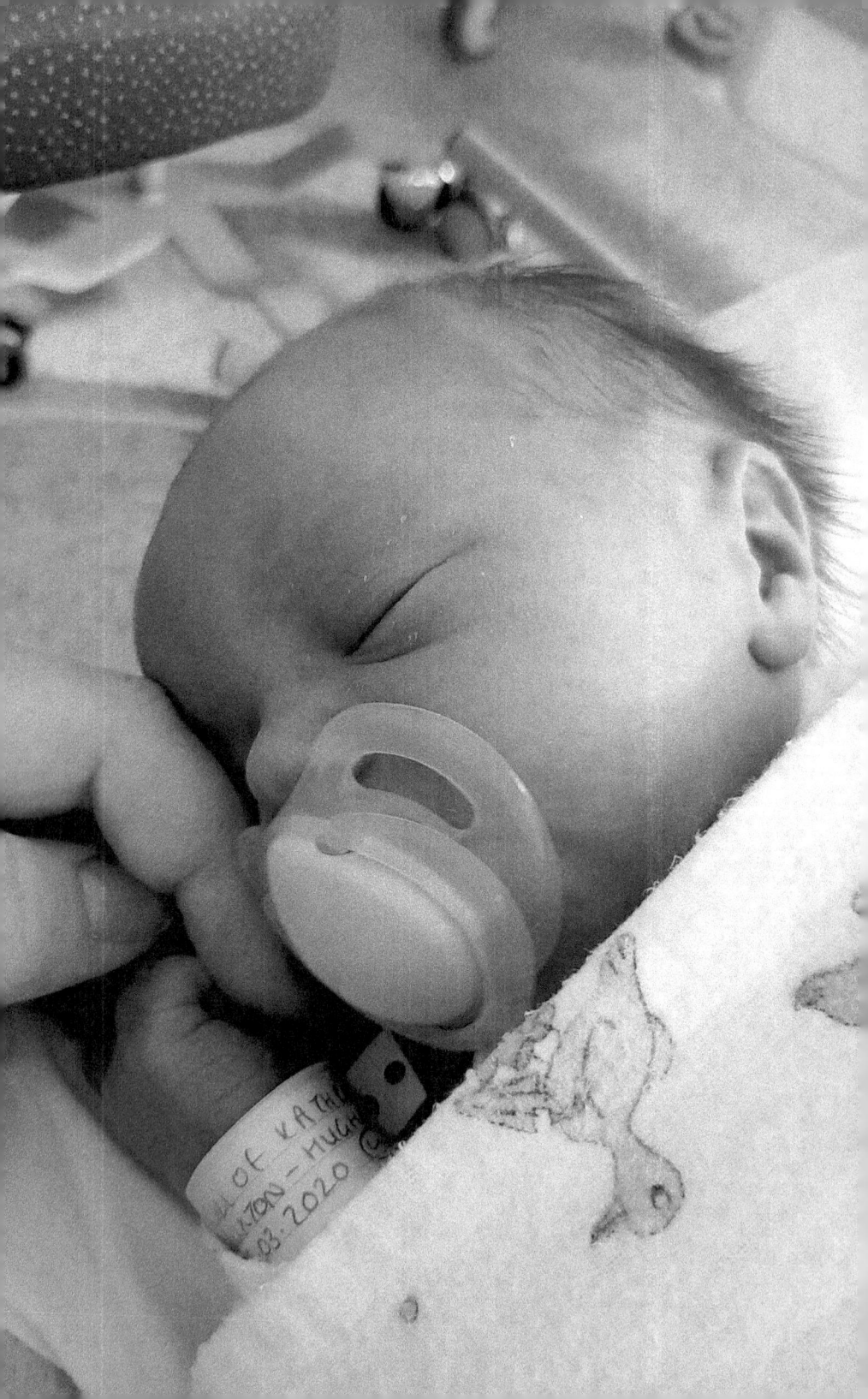

No. 18

Kathryn's Story

My daughter was due March 30th and at first it was an exciting time for my family. However, at week 33 I was admitted to Glangwili for reduced fetal movement, and during a follow up growth scan it was discovered that my baby wasn't growing properly anymore. Week 35 showed little change in her weight again and we were starting to worry. At week 37 we had our third growth scan and once again her weight hadn't changed. In fact, it had now fallen off the chart!

I was sent to Carmarthen Hospital on the 11th March from the appointment in Withybush Hospital. The plan was to induce me, and it very quickly became a stressful time. The virus was just starting to rear its head in the UK but at the time it was the least of our worries. Aside from plenty of hand sanitiser on the antenatal ward, nothing seemed too different.

We tried various methods of induction over three days, but nothing worked. Eventually I was taken for an emergency caesarean in the early hours of 15th March. My daughter was born a tiny 5lb 4oz (spot on the scan estimates) at 00:44, at 37+6 weeks. My mum and my husband both got to meet her before I was taken down to the post-natal ward. The plan was for them and other family members to come up to the hospital over the next few days to meet her.

However, later that morning the Head of Midwifery made the decision to close the ward to all visitors, to prevent the spread of the coronavirus. This meant my family couldn't come to the hospital, and my husband had to stay home to look after his eldest daughter.

My baby needed to be taken to the Special Care Baby Unit as she couldn't keep her blood sugar up. I felt as though I had failed my Baby, and it was horrible to be separated from her. I couldn't stay with her at first because the Special Care Baby Unit was too busy, so I was sent back to the ward without my Baby. The other three women on the ward all had their babies with them and I felt so alone.

I didn't have any family members to support me, so it was a very difficult time. The Midwives were lovely about it, but they aren't family so it's never the same. As a sleep deprived new mum my hormones were all over the place and not having that support of family except for over the phone, it was truly horrible.

Seeing my daughter hooked up to machines with a tube in her nose was heart-breaking, and I couldn't talk to anyone about it because they couldn't be there with me. She spent 24 hours there and the day that they discharged her back to me, they decided that it was too risky to have non-medical staff on the ward. Had she been admitted any later I wouldn't have been able to be with her at all and that would have been incredibly hard to cope with.

My husband was eventually able to get to the hospital on Monday, but it was very hard not having my family able to come and meet my baby. It felt very isolating.

There was a funny feeling on the ward, as if people were starting to worry about the virus. The Midwives did an excellent job at staying calm and following hygiene procedures. They weren't wearing masks, visors or aprons at the time, so it still felt familiar. I feel lucky that I was also able to share a room with three other women, so I did still have some company, but it wasn't the same.

When we were discharged from hospital on the 18th March the hospital was in the process of closing to all visitors.

We had Midwives out to our home twice once we were discharged. Once the day after we came home and once for the 5-day check. After that the Midwife was meant to take over, but she couldn't come out. She was meant to call every week, but they were too thinly stretched.

My daughter struggled to keep milk down for the first week and she struggled with a poor latch due to tongue tie and just being so small. She also had a horrible nappy rash that quickly got out of hand. We tried to call the midwives or the health visitors so they could advise, but it was impossible to get through to either of them. It was stressful and scary and there were many tears shed. My husband and I also had our six-year-old to look after, so we were stretched pretty thin. Our families could only offer advice over the phone.

We weren't able to get my daughter weighed until she was Eight weeks old. Thankfully, she had gained plenty of weight but there were many times I contemplated giving up on breastfeeding because I just didn't have any help or support. Thankfully, everything was okay, and we worked out breastfeeding and eventually sorted her nappy.

My childbirth was a scary one and quite upsetting emotionally. I was lucky that my husband was still able to come and visit us but being in hospital when the virus was starting to seriously affect the country was scary. I would think twice before having another baby as the experience still upsets me now.

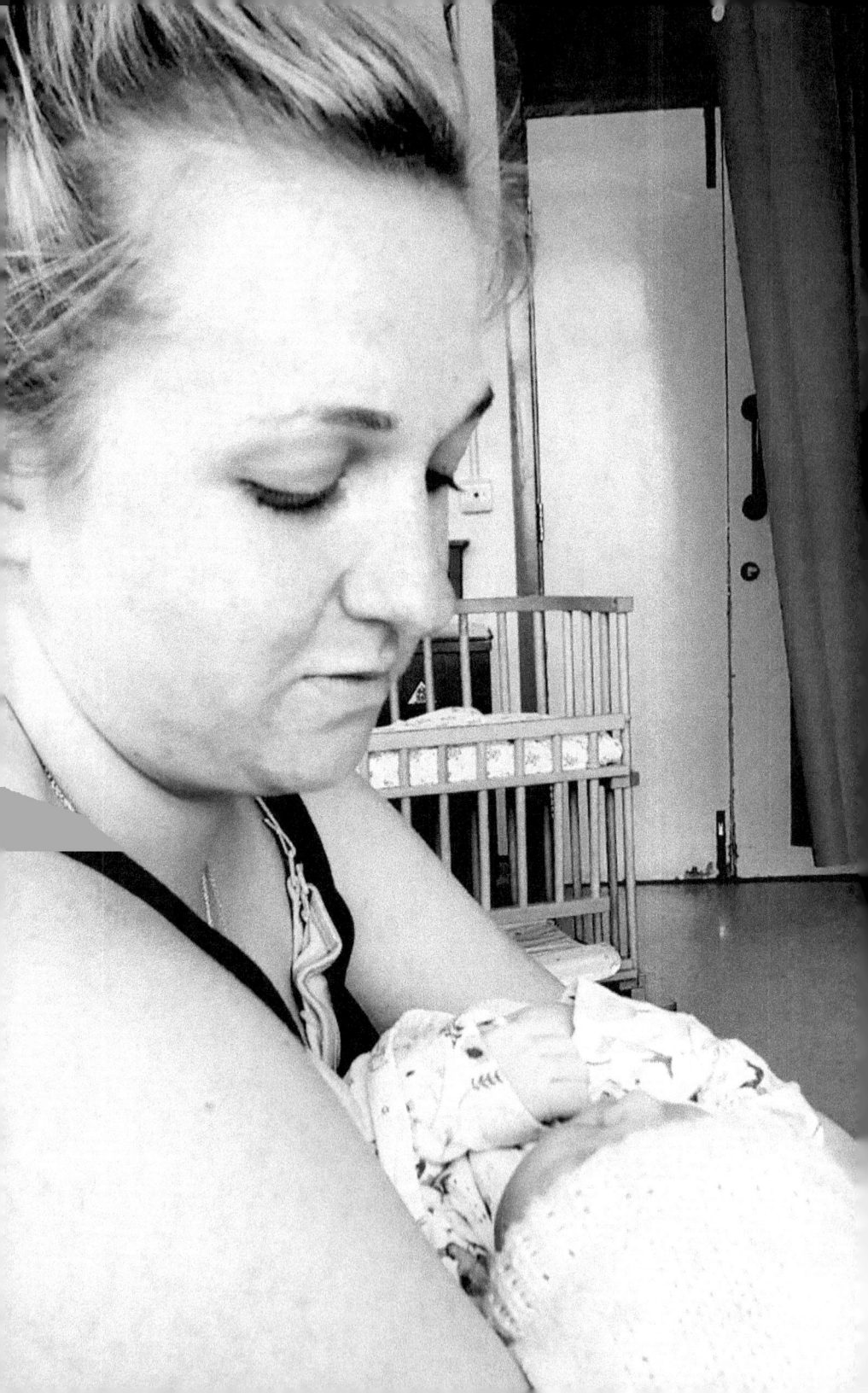

No. 19
Megan's Story

So, I also have a 2-and-a-half-year-old who wasn't born during a pandemic so its great comparison.

Emily was born on 13/4/20. Everything was normal until I was 36 weeks pregnant and pregnant women were now classed as high risk, so I went on maternity leave a week early (luckily).

I started suffering with extreme anxiety because my husband was working in the leisure centre industry and was coming into contact with a lot of people.(I have a history of slight anxiety and depression) at 37 weeks I noticed reduced movements, I went and for movement tracing monitoring, I had to go by myself (which causes even more stress because you are already worried) but the Midwife was lovely and kept me calm.

I was supposed to have a growth scan at 38 weeks , but because I was low risk and only consultant led because of my mother's history, I had to make the very difficult decision to not go (I spoke with many health professionals to help me make this decision) but I should not have had to make this decision , and it may have picked up that Emily was in a funny position and so she got a bit stuck. But we will never know. I scheduled an appointment with the Midwife to make sure everything was ok, and it was but we had to use our cars as waiting areas, and be called in one by one, again by myself. By this point we were in full lockdown and my husband wasn't in work anymore, but I wasn't allowed to see my mum and have her support which was awful.

I then started to panic, what if I wasn't allowed a birth partner at all? My husband had a breakdown over Christmas, and I was worried that missing the birth if his child would set him back mentally again. Who was going to look after my toddler while I was in labour? Would I be safe coming home to my toddler after being in hospital? Along with all the other worries like how to get food and keep my toddler busy!

So, we started going for very long walks every day which I'm sure helped my labour progress so quickly!

I had a Midwife appointment at 39 weeks and expressed I was worried about birth anyway and I was worried that I wouldn't be able to have a birth partner and so was my husband. She said that they were really going to try to avoid this. She also explained that the Midwives would be wearing full personal protective clothing during the birth and it would be strange anyway. This didn't really bother me (I felt sorry for the Midwives) because for everyone to stay safe was a priority!

So I went into labour a few days early and it was very quick, I stayed at home a bit longer than I should have because I thought the longer I stay at home the less at risk I still be.

So when I phoned to ask to come down I was told I had to find the new ward by myself, I got lost and a man who had seen me at the door showed me where to go, I was crying and in pain. My temperature was checked when I got there, and the Midwives were wearing masks. They were so sweet and still managed to calm me down, my husband was then rushed in, she could tell it was all happening quite fast, his temperature was checked. Although I was well looked after and felt safe, the whole time, I could feel them rushing and getting everything ready especially because they had to put extra PPE to put on. I had my heart set on an epidural, but I most definitely didn't have time for one of those! I got to hospital about 5 am and I was 7cm and she was out by 6:06!

So, he was allowed to stay for a few hours which was lovely, and I managed to have a wash and get sorted. My husband was just pleased he got to be at the birth and managed to spend a few hours with his new daughter, but he was sad he had to leave, luckily we had our eldest daughter for him to go home to and keep him entertained!

I definitely felt the covid 19 situation when I got moved up to the ward, (because Emily had pooped I had to stay overnight) the only interaction I got was when checks were made or food was brought to me (I understood this was for everyone's safety) everyone was still lovely but I felt very lonely and like the magic had been taken away from what had just happened, I had no one to talk to, or celebrate with, and I felt very sad . Then we had the most horrendous first night, as she was unsettled, I was so upset. The Midwife was lovely, and so caring and helped very much as Emily and I were both very distressed. By the morning I was almost hysterical at the thought of not going home to get some help and support from my husband and see my eldest daughter. After having all the checks, we were sent home.

I felt very sad that the last few weeks of my pregnancy were shadowed with such uncertainty and anxiety. I am very sad that I didn't have anyone to celebrate the birth of my daughter with. I was very pleased with the level of care that was provided, even though I'm sure the Midwives were under a lot of pressure and stress themselves. And the Personal protective clothing didn't bother me at all.

The support after giving birth and getting

home hasn't really affected me, I've still had many phone calls, and I have been able to get any support that I have needed, And I have very much liked not having to share my baby with anyone, or get dressed and tidy the house for visitors!

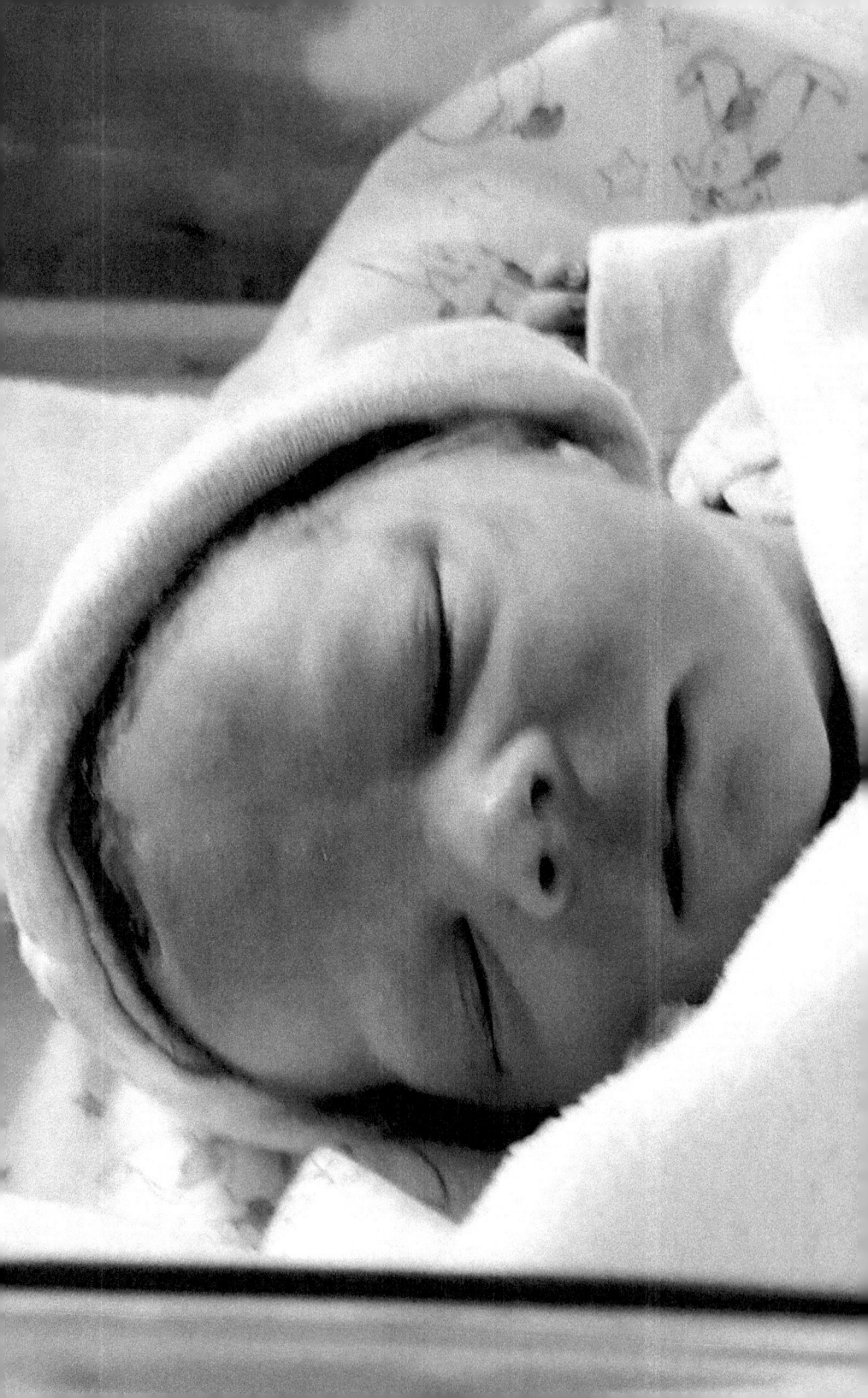

No. 20

Kath's Story

I am 41 years old and I became pregnant in 2019 and was already a little anxious as I had a miscarriage in November 2018 at almost eleven weeks. We therefore paid for an early pregnancy scan to check progress, this was normal and showed that I was six weeks pregnant so provided some reassurances, however I felt in denial, a defensive mechanism I believe.

We kept the pregnancy a secret until after the dating scan and then shared our news with close friends and work as a necessity for risk assessment purposes. I was given a due date of the 17th of March 2020. The anomaly scan was also normal, but I still felt a little nervous and uncertain. I attended my routine antenatal appointments and everything was going well until on one appointment my midwife measured me small for dates, an ultra sound scan was arranged the following day which measured me large for dates and I had to attend for a glucose tolerance test at the end of that week.

The GTT was done on the 23rd of January and came back slightly elevated and I was then treated for gestational diabetes, I found this very hard to accept initially as it made a massive difference I really didn't want to end up with an induction. My diabetes was monitored and managed with diet alone, I was seen weekly in diabetic clinic and attended for growth scans. I first became aware of coronavirus around mid-February when the spread to Italy was publicised and at this point, I suppose I was quite ignorant to the impact that it was going to have.

On the 4th of March at 38 weeks I attended for a scan and then clinic, the scan showed that there was a reduction in growth and the consultant was concerned and arranged for an induction the following day. The Midwife in clinic gave me a sweep in order to hopefully start labour without the need for induction. Overnight I began to experience contractions and I attended the hospital as planned the following day, no induction medications were required as I was in labour, my waters were broken, and Charlie was born later that day. We had to stay in hospital as Charlie was on the hypoglycaemia pathway. On Saturday the 7th of March while awaiting discharge it became obvious that coronavirus was going to impact on our lives.

The panic buying of toilet rolls, hand sanitizer and hand soap had already begun prior to this but now there were even more concerns. When I was discharged, we had some visitors at home however this was limited as the spread of the virus was at the forefront of everyone's minds. I had most of my postnatal midwifery care without any problems this only changed for the Health visitors first visit and my midwifery discharge, on both occasions I received phone calls to check whether anyone in the house was symptomatic. They both attended wearing gloves and aprons and did not touch anything, the Health visitor weighed Charlie that day (I handled him and put him on and off the scales) and he hasn't been weighed since he is now 12 weeks old.

When Charlie was two weeks old we noticed a firm lump on the right side of his neck just below his ear, I rang the health visitor who said that she would usually advise to attend the GP's however due to corona virus to keep an eye on it as it was likely to be a swollen gland. A week went by and with no improvement I rang the GP, an appointment was arranged that day, the GP couldn't find any cause for infection so discussed with paediatrics who advised to observe for another week rather than risk exposure in hospital.

Another week went by with no change and so we attended the hospital for review, at this time I was scared of what the findings might be, my husband was furloughed but only one of us could attend appointments due to the restrictions. I felt alone and unsupported during our attendance to hospital although the staff despite being behind masks were friendly and accommodating. Following an ultrasound scan of his neck Charlie was diagnosed with torticollis a knot in the muscle of his neck which was reassuring. All further consultation with physiotherapy and consultants has been via telephone, this has been difficult when explaining exercises to perform with Charlie and the absence of demonstration however the lump has gone now.

Having a baby during this pandemic has had a massive impact on Charlie's first few months, there are friends and family who haven't met him yet, he hasn't been held by anyone except me, his dad and his sister, this concerns me whether be will have a bond with his grandparents. I am anxious regarding my return to work and the length of time we will be in isolation as Charlie isn't familiar with anyone else, so this is likely to be stressful for him. I have had to attend all his appointments on my own, which has been very difficult and upsetting on occasions.

I have missed out on weighing him, attending mother and toddler and breastfeeding groups although I have made use of the breastfeeding helpline! When I had my daughter (17 years ago!!) I returned to work six weeks after her birth so felt like I missed out on the support groups so was excited to attend this time, it seems it's not meant to be. Rather than being able to meet with other mothers and health professionals I have had to research things myself and I have felt that I question everything I do without this additional support.

Being isolated I suppose has also had its benefits, I have had an uninterrupted time with my baby and despite some tough times we now have breastfeeding well established. Even though he hasn't been weighed I can see he is thriving, and we do try to weigh him on our scales. Overall, I have enjoyed having Charlie to myself although I am concerned for the future.

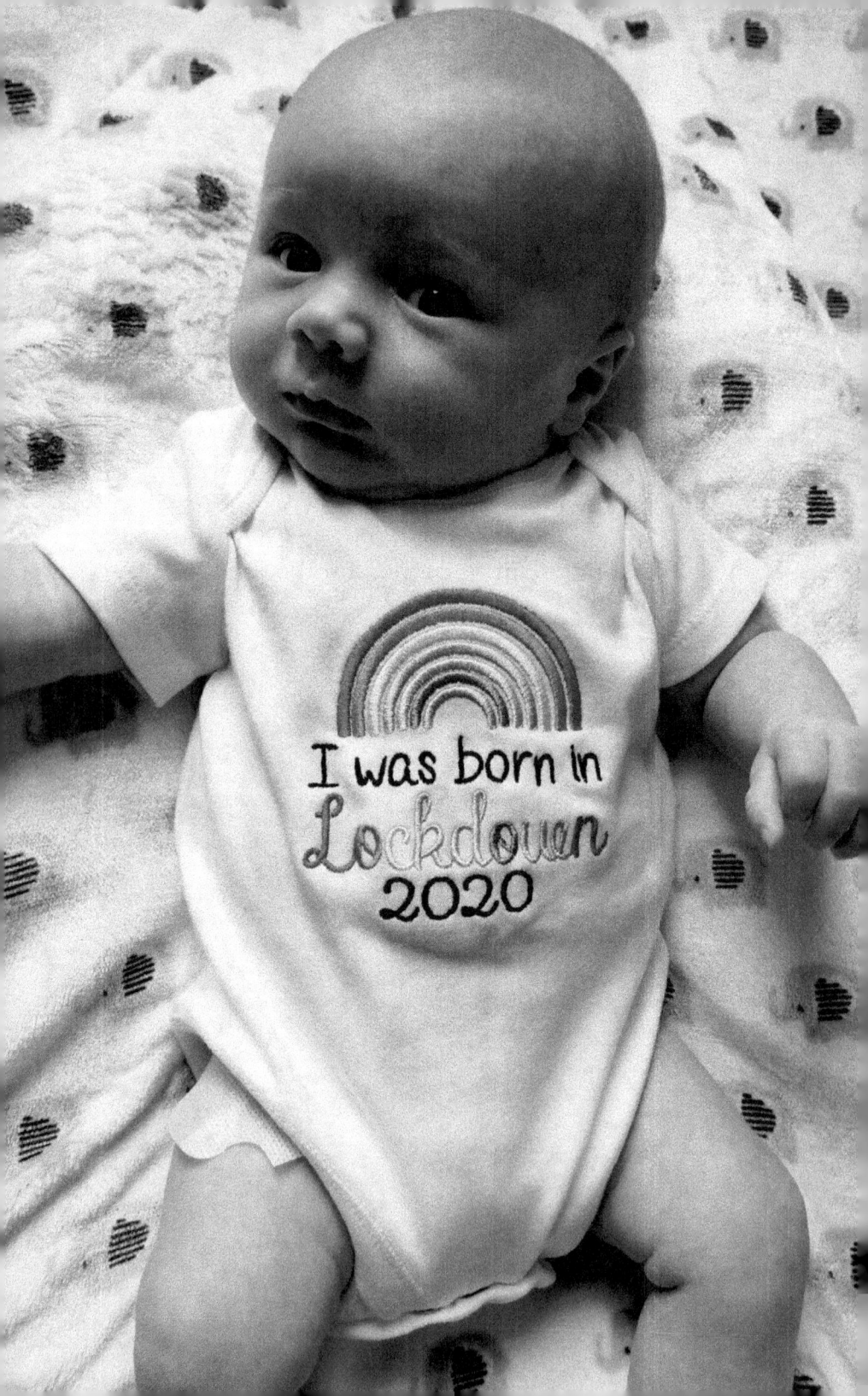

No. 21

Kath J's Story

We are a family of four, I live with my partner, Rich, and two children, Emelia 17 months and Toby, 4 weeks old.

My personal worries about the corona virus were heightened when pregnant women were put on the "at risk" category. At this time, I was 34 weeks pregnant. To hear I was on the at-risk category was very scary. My instant reaction was to worry about how the virus would put my unborn baby at risk. I started my maternity leave two weeks early and we pulled Emelia out of nursery straight away. Emelia and I self-isolated at home. Rich is a key worker and was going to work every day. This was a worry for us but couldn't be avoided.

This was a very difficult situation as I was heavily pregnant and caring for Emelia by myself. In normal circumstances Emelia would spend time at nursery and I would have a lot of help from family. It was difficult for Emelia because she was used to being busy, going to parks, seeing other children and family. Instead we stayed at home for six weeks before Toby arrived.

I attended two antenatal appointments at Prince Phillip Hospital during this time. I was told I had to attend the appointments alone. As this was my second baby, I wasn't too worried about this as I felt I knew what to expect. I was nervous about going into the hospital, after spending so many weeks at home. I felt there was a risk being around other people. There were social distancing measures in place at the hospital, but this didn't ease my anxiety. At my first appointment the consultant told me to prepare for the possibility of Rich not being able to be at the birth. I was having a planned caesarean section and the thought of going through this alone was very scary. I was really upset and worried. This was around the same time as field hospitals were being built as the NHS was expecting such high numbers of covid patients. This terrified me as I was imagining hospitals being full of extremely sick patients. I was worried about the newborn picking up the virus whilst we were in hospital.

After this appointment I spoke to my Community Midwife who told me as things stand partners can attend the birth but will not be able to visit on the ward afterwards. However, no one could predict how things would be around the time I was due to have my baby.

We also had the added worry of who was going to care for Emelia if both of us were at the birth. We had not seen family or friends since the beginning of lockdown. As my Mum lived alone and also isolating, we made the decision that she could look after Emelia at our house whilst Rich was with me for the birth.

Closer to my due date I was informed that Rich could be at the birth and spend some time with me and the baby to settle us in on the ward afterwards. I was also told as long as baby and I am well we could go home the next day. Under these circumstances I was happy with this as I understood this had to happen so all mums and babies on the ward could be kept as safe as possible.

I went into Glangwili hospital as planned on the 27th April to have our baby via caesarean section. When we arrived at the ward the Midwives took both mine and Rich's temperatures and asked if we had any Covid symptoms. As we were both well, we went onto the ward. The Midwives were very friendly and put me at ease. The atmosphere on the ward felt completely normal. My focus was on the birth and having a healthy baby and I was able to switch off from my worries over the virus. The caesarean section went well, and our healthy baby boy was delivered that morning. As I wasn't feeling very well after the section Rich was able to stay with me on the ward until I was settled and ready for him to leave. I didn't have any pressure from the Midwives for him to leave before I was ready. We chose to close the curtains and have a few hours getting to know our baby boy Toby, in private. When Rich left, we were told he then wouldn't be allowed back in to visit. When I was ready to leave, he would have to meet me at the entrance of the hospital. Having to look after Toby alone after having the caesarean section was very difficult. The Midwives helped as much as they could, but they were very busy. The next afternoon both Toby and I were checked by the Consultant and were told we could go home. The Midwives helped us down to the hospital entrance where we met Rich.

Toby is now five weeks old. It's been a very special but surreal five weeks. We've been fortunate to have so much time as a family of four and have enjoyed our little bubble. However, it's also been very upsetting that our family and friends haven't been able to meet Toby. Our family and close friends have visited to see Toby and chat through our window. This has been so hard for Grandparents, Aunties and Uncles who I know would love to hold him and get to know him properly.

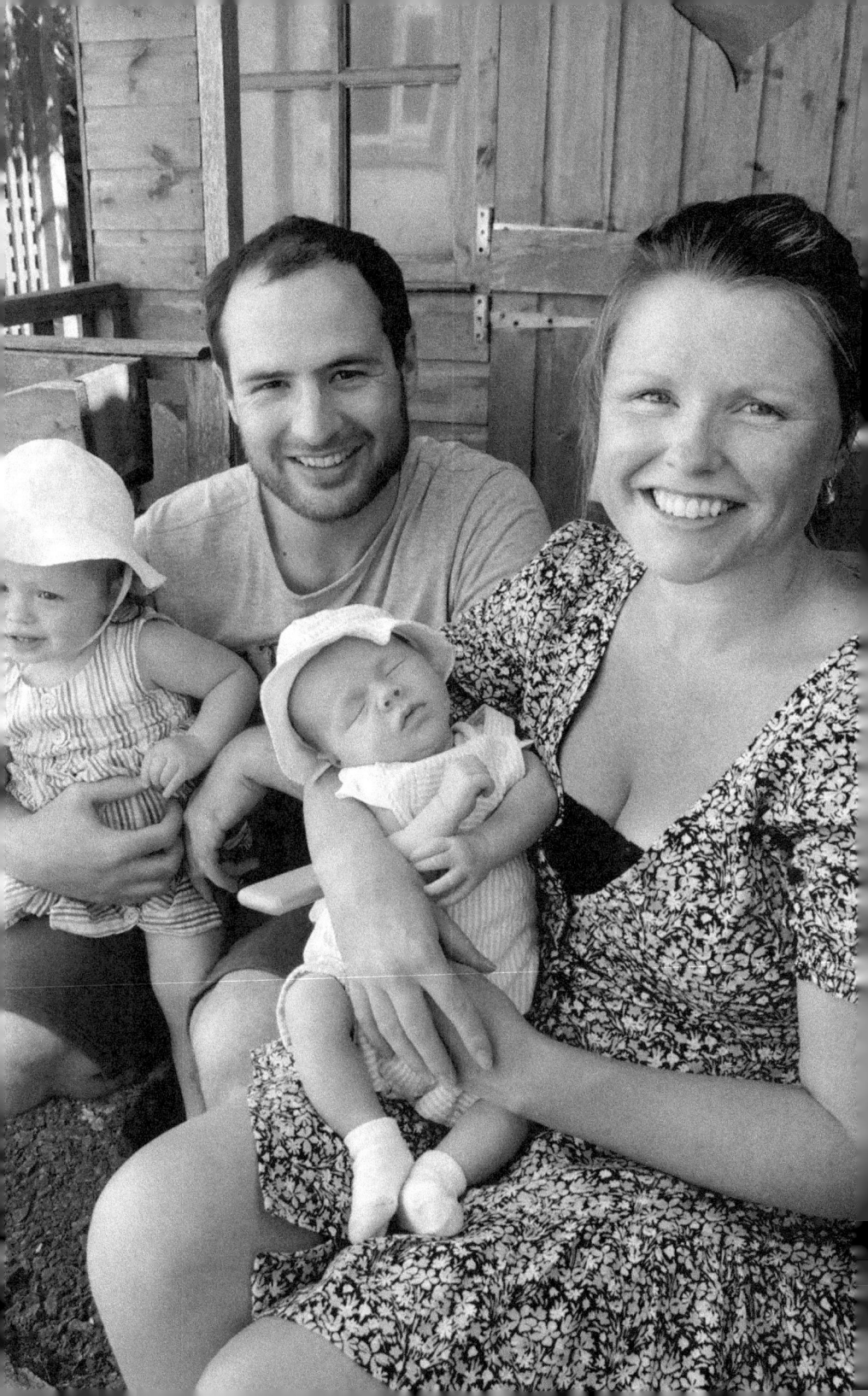

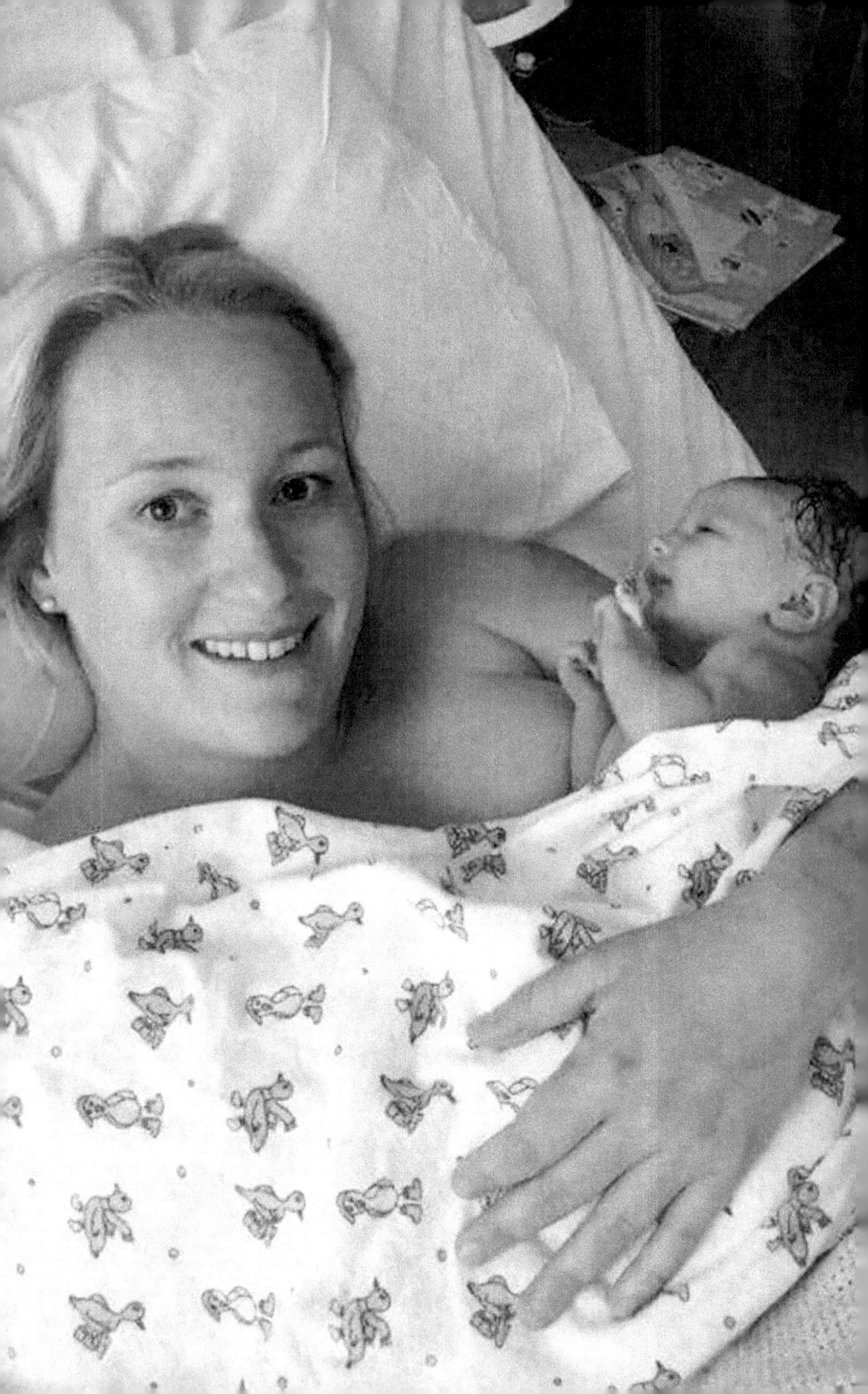

No. 22
Rosie's Story

I delivered my first born in February 2018 in the Midwife Led Unit and had a wonderful water birth. It was the best thing ever. When she was eight months old, I had a very nasty fall and suffered a subdural haematoma and had brain surgery in Cardiff. I was off work for seven months and unable to drive for eight months. I was very lucky to fully recover and the only thing I have to remember is my complete loss of smell, which in fact when you have a newborn and a toddler it does help not being able to smell their nappies!!

When I found out I was expecting in the September we were over the moon and excited to have something to focus on and take our minds off the past year which had been challenging after my fall. This time the Midwives decided I needed Consultant led care to ensure I was fully supported throughout the pregnancy. In my first appointment with the Consultant I was quite anxious as we talked about my head injury and if we thought it could affect birth. We discussed a few options, perhaps a natural birth would put too much pressure on my brain. We also chatted about a caesarean. Luckily, my Consultant from the Heath was in touch and said because it was a traumatic brain injury and not an acquired brain injury, she didn't see any reason why I could not give birth naturally. This was all before we'd even heard of Covid-19.

When I was 29 weeks pregnant Boris Johnson added pregnant women to the vulnerable category. This is when things began to change. I didn't see the Midwife personally between 28 and 37 weeks. However, I had spoken to them on the phone and was reassured at any point if there was a problem or a query to feel I could ring them anytime. Luckily, my pregnancy was great, and I didn't need to ring them. I continued to see my Consultant monthly which was great as they measured my bump and listened to baby's heartbeat. My Consultant was very happy with me and handed me back to Midwife Led Care at 37 weeks.

When I was 39 weeks pregnant I had quite a big bleed and passed a clot. I was very scared and rang Glangwili Hospital immediately, I just thought the worst. They were fantastic and very reassuring on the phone, they suggested I left as soon as possible to come in to be examined. By this point I knew my husband wouldn't be allowed in with me, he took me to the door and the Midwife and Health Care Assistant greeted me. I was taken to a bed and hooked up to the monitoring machine straight away.

The Midwife had asked me was the baby moving normally, I was worrying so much about the bleed I hadn't noticed if the baby had moved at all. My mind was put at ease straight away with the machine showing that baby was very happy and moving, my blood pressure and heart rate also normal. It was the best feeling to know that our baby was healthy. Even though the baby was happy the Doctor decided to keep me in for the night to be monitored. The care from the staff on the antenatal ward was amazing - from the cleaners to the consultants, all very friendly and welcoming. The whole 24 hrs or so that I was in I didn't even remember about Covid, nothing was mentioned. The staff were in masks, but by this point it wasn't really anything new to me as was used to seeing the staff in masks from my Midwife and Consultant appointments. I was then discharged the following morning, by this point the consultant on the ward said I was to give birth on the Labour ward and not MLU after my head injury and bleed. This came as a shock as even though I had accepted there were no water births I had hoped for a natural birth in the MLU. The Midwife reassured me and said not to worry, perhaps I wouldn't be hooked up to the monitor the whole time etc.

When I was home, I was getting more anxious about the birth being on the labour ward. I had a Skype call with the Consultant Midwife, she was fantastic and after our chat she didn't see any reason why I couldn't give birth naturally in the MLU and wrote a letter to confirm this for my notes.

My due date was Monday June 1st. The morning of the 4th I wasn't sure if my waters had gone or was it discharge linked to the bleed I'd had. I rang my community midwife and as I had an appointment booked that day anyway, she said not to worry, and they would take a swab there to test if it was waters or not. My appointment was at 1:40, she did the antenatal checks and then I had the test to see if it was waters. As I got up from the bed, I had a gush, and there they were - my waters!! I apologised to the midwife! And asked for some tissue to clean the floor!! My contractions started straight away around 2pm and it wasn't long before they were very close together.

We arrived at the antenatal ward at around 5:45pm on Thursday June 4th. I was really well looked after straight away by two midwives. After being examined and 5cm dilated I was able to ring my husband to come and join me. The contractions were coming very strong and quickly at this point. The whole team on the ward worked very hard to get the labour room ready for me as they had only just discharged a lady and my contractions were so strong, we knew it wouldn't be much longer.

The senior Midwife was amazing, she even rubbed my back throughout the contractions and kept telling me how well I was doing. As soon as they were kitted out in their full PPE (they had to rush as baby was coming!) our little daughter Cadi Mair was born at 7:16pm weighing 7lbs2. The senior Midwife popped in at the end of her shift to see how labour was progressing and was shocked to see Cadi had arrived!

Straight after labour I had a high temperature 38.1, the Midwives were a little worried. They suggested I had a bath, opened windows to cool down and they would take it again in an hour. This was the first time I heard the word coronavirus. The Midwife said if my temperature didn't decrease, I would have to be moved to the red zone and be tested. This was heart-breaking to hear but I did understand it was all to follow protocol. Luckily after an hour my temperature dropped, and we were discharged about 12:30am. The night shift Midwife arranged for the Community Midwives to come out and do the newborn checks the next day. An absolutely amazing experience at Glangwili Hospital yet again.

The Community Midwife came to the house the following day to check Cadi over. She then booked us an appointment for the heel prick on day five in Tenby Cottage Hospital. With my first born the heel prick was done at the house, but I know with the current situation the Midwives are trying to avoid too many house calls if possible. I have to be honest; it was really lovely to leave the house!

We all went in the car, and then after the appointment we had a lovely walk as a family of four. The Midwife then phoned me on day ten to check how Cadi was doing and of course how I was doing. It was lovely to chat to her and just touch base. She was happy with everything and discharged us.

To conclude, even though this weird, unknown situation we are all currently in, the care I have received before birth, during and after has been fantastic. All the staff have looked after myself and Cadi extremely well and I am forever grateful to them.

Thank you!

Rosie's Story

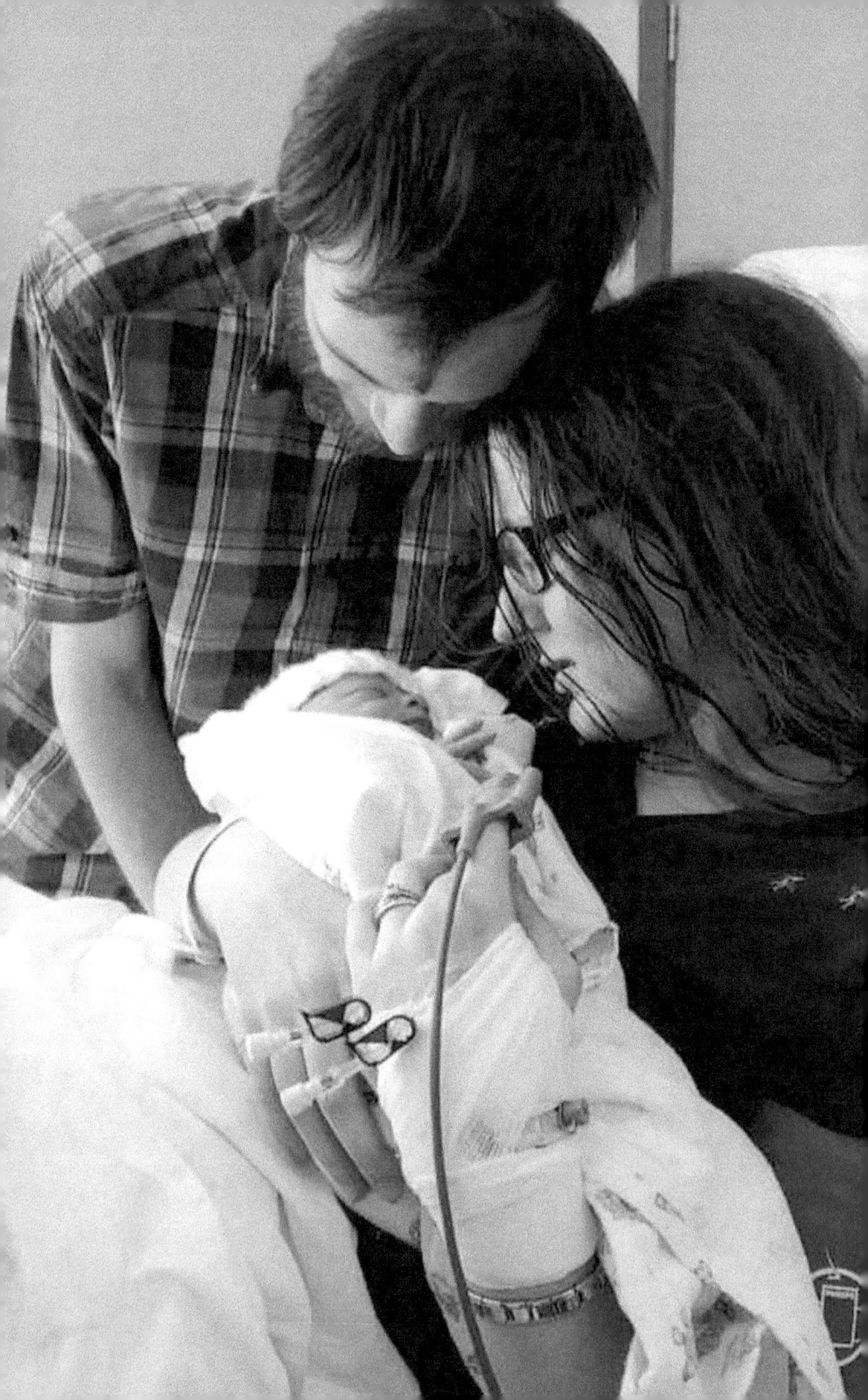

No. 23
Vicky's Story

We found out we were having our third baby in November 2019. It was a very anxious time for us as we had sadly had a loss earlier in the year so naturally, we had anxieties seeing a positive test. We had some issues early on which increased our worries but by our twenty- week scan everything seemed perfect and we found we were having another boy!

The excitement started to kick in from that point. I was told I'd have regular growth scans from 28 weeks due to a previous premature birth and two IUGR babies. (Intra uterine growth retardation).

We weren't too worried when we first heard about coronavirus, we had the very naive attitude of "oh it's just like the flu" so didn't worry too much as were young and healthy. Once other countries started to lockdown and the number of cases in the UK went up, we quickly realised this wasn't just the flu and took it much more seriously. We both have numerous high risk family members so we worried for them more than ourselves and when it's was announced that pregnant women were considered high risk it did start to panic us as there was so little info about if it affected babies in the womb and all I seemed to see on social media was horror stories and the awful few cases where pregnant women or newborn babies were critically ill.

My anxiety really peaked from then on and once lockdown was announced we took it very seriously. It hugely affected our two- year -old, not being able to see my husband friends and family and not being able to go to nursery but we explained best we could and tried not to show our worries to him.

My growth scans started at roughly this time and not having my husband there did put a downer on it but the staff were all extra lovely even given all the pressure they were under and my 28 week scan went amazing and I didn't feel so anxious going to my 32 week scan. We were told from this point that my baby wasn't growing well and that I had reduced amniotic fluid so I would need weekly scans and monitoring to keep an eye on things.

These appointments always worried me because it felt like another thing going wrong. I'm still very much grieving for our son who passed away last year so hearing our baby was doing anything less than amazing really was tough for me. This is when having to go alone to appointments really got to me and I almost started to dread them. My husband felt very left out although he totally understood and agreed with every rule that was in place and he's felt a little detached from the whole experience. At 37 weeks my Consultant told me my baby had dropped to the 3rd Growth centile and that it was best to induce me. She gave me a date for the 3rd July, just two days -time. I left the appointment both excited and absolutely terrified. I had to try explaining it all to my partner when I still couldn't get my own head around it all. We had a lot to sort out, so it was pretty much panic stations now we had been given a date.

I got to the hospital at 2.30pm on June 3rd. We had stopped for a KFC on the way as they'd opened back up a few days before, so we ate that in the car and then my husband helped me carry my bags to Dinefwr ward. I had to say goodbye to him at the doors and a Midwife took me to the ward. I felt like crying because my husband couldn't be with me and as it was an induction, we had no idea how long I would be in hospital for. It was also the first time leaving my son in over twelve weeks and he was really playing on my mind.

A Midwife brought over a monitor and set it all up and said she would be back after reading my notes. She came back at 5pm and examined me. I was 1cm but my cervix was thick, so she decided to insert the twenty-four-hour pessary and explained the process to me. I went back on the monitor for half an hour and the trace was perfect, so I decided to ring my husband before trying to get some sleep. I was feeling really homesick but started talking to the other lady in the ward who was lovely, and it helped speed up some of the time.

Through the night I was having irregular tightenings but not a lot happened. In the morning the pains were getting more painful but were still irregular. I asked for a ball to bounce on and they started getting more regular. At 10am I asked if the Midwife would examine me, I was 3cm but there wasn't space on labour ward so she decided not to pop my waters yet but left the pessary in place so it could finish thinning my cervix.

By 12pm the pain was getting really intense, so I was put on a monitor for 15 minutes. The monitor was showing that I was having contractions every 2-3 minutes, so the midwife decided to examine me again. I was 7cm, and my waters were bulging so I got taken to labour ward. I rung my husband straight away, as we lived 30 minutes away and my two previous labours were very fast. I was really worried that he would miss the birth. I got to labour ward at 12.45pm and had two lovely Midwives with me.

The Midwife explained they were going to get a doctor to insert a cannula in case I haemorrhaged again, and she offered me gas and air. I was calm during my contractions and they supported me while we waited for my husband to arrive. It didn't phase me that they were wearing ppe, it made it feel safer for me and them, even though the virus wasn't ever a thought, the entire time. My husband arrived around 1.15pm and I had been having the urge to push for a few minutes' prior, but my waters were still intact. I felt so relived seeing my husband and the pain almost instantly intensified, and I began pushing. At 1.49pm my baby was born. He had the usual level of care and all the checks were done. It took a while for the placenta to come out, but the staff did a great job of getting my husband involved with the baby. We knew he would have to leave soon so I'm glad he still got to dress and feed the baby and have some time with us.

We had to stay overnight due to him being small, he needed to have his blood sugar levels checked before we could go home. The Midwives we had back on the Postnatal Ward were amazing. I felt great after the birth so could do everything for the baby and didn't need a lot of help, but the amount of breastfeeding support I had was incredible. I was shown how to cup feed, hand express and they were more than happy to check the latch was right. We quickly noticed that he had a tongue tie which was affecting feeding but by the morning the staff had already put a referral in place for it to be snipped once we were discharged. All the staff were amazing again and nothing seemed like too much of a problem for them. A Midwife even offered to wash the baby's hair for me which was a huge help! The ward was really busy, so it took hours for us to be discharged but I totally understood the pressure the staff were under.

We got discharged at 6.30pm and went straight to get the baby's tongue tie snipped. The staff saw to him quickly and we were on the way home. We had to pick-up our son from my parents' house, so they did meet the baby at the same time, but they are the only ones that have met him so far.

A big worry I'd had was that lockdown wouldn't be lifted before my baby was born and due to my anxieties from our middle son passing away, I wanted the baby to meet everyone straight away in case the worst happened again and we lost him too. Sadly, due to lockdown everyone is going to have to wait until it's over to meet him and we have no idea how long that will be, but we focus on the positive that we get to be in our bubble of just the four of us and get that quality time together.

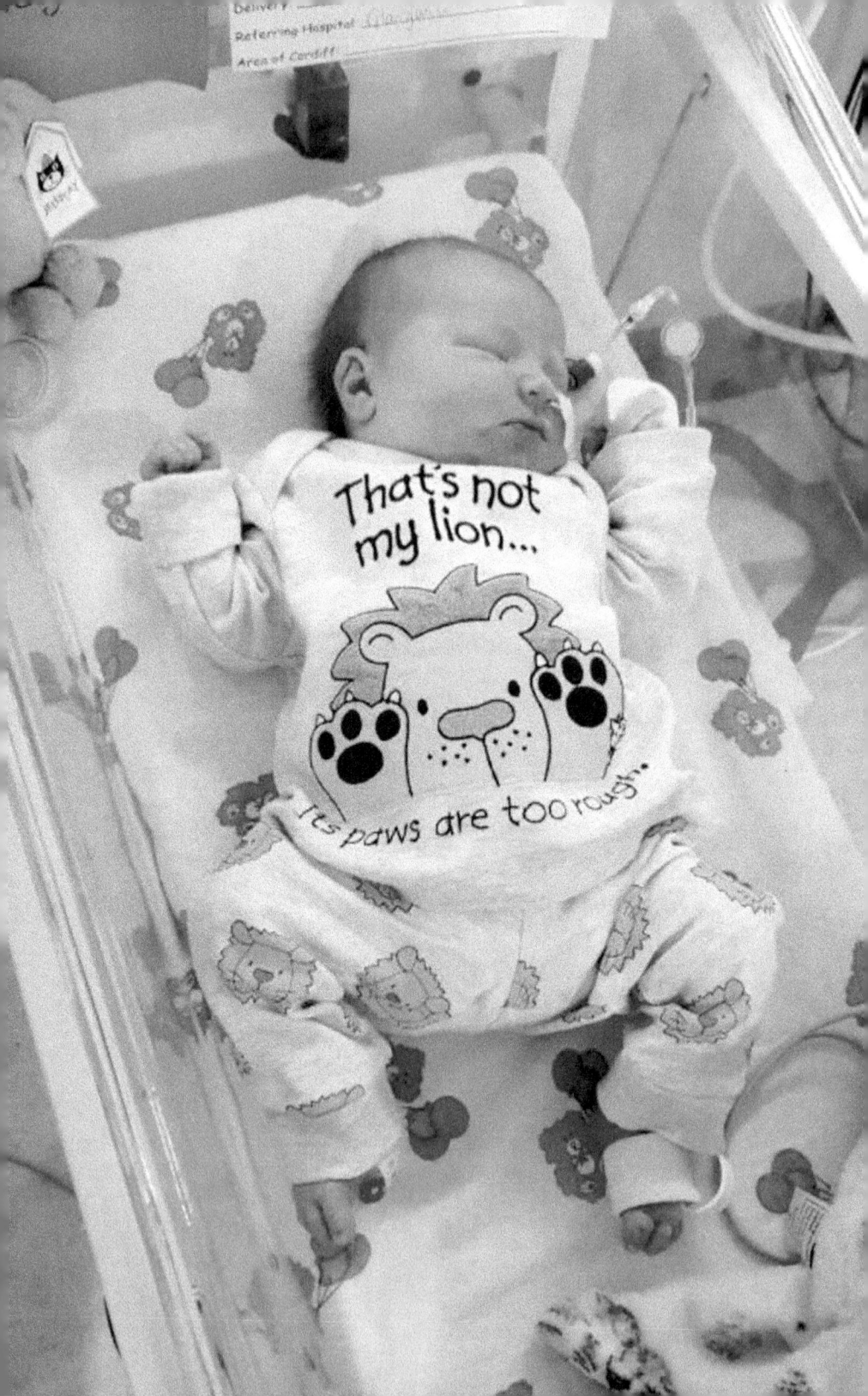

No. 24

Samantha's Story

We found out we were pregnant last year before it all began, by the time coronavirus had taken over I was seven months pregnant, the last two months were hard, I was heavily pregnant with Gestational Diabetes and the baby was growing large, so regular check- ups were needed. It was difficult not being able to take my husband to appointments with me, but the staff were lovely and always made me feel at ease.

My Consultant examined me at 38 weeks and said it was best for me to deliver my baby via elective caesarean section as the baby's weight gain was increasing rapidly due to the Gestational Diabetes, so, that was it, my baby had been given her eviction date, Ha ha!!.

When I was going in for my planned caesarean-section I wasn't worried as the staff had all been so good, I knew I had nothing to worry about.

On Tuesday 12th May my partner and I arrived at hospital at 8.30am. We were welcomed by the friendly and caring staff and taken to the bed to get ready to meet our princess. At 9.30am I was taken to theatre. The Midwife accompanying me was amazing and reassured me the whole time. The theatre staff were very thorough and explained everything as it was happening.

I felt safe and well informed about what was going to happen. Baby Griffiths was born at safely at 10.31am weighing 9lb 6oz. During her birth check the Midwife noticed a problem with her back passage. Baby was placed in my arms and we were taken back to ward to begin recovery. The baby needed to be transferred to the Heath in Cardiff for an assessment by the specialist team up there. The staff on ward were so caring and reassuring. The baby was taken to the Special Care Baby Unit SCBU) and incubated ready for transfer. I was never once worried as I could tell the Midwives cared for my baby as much as I did. Nothing was ever too much trouble and once my husband had left to go to Cardiff to be with baby the Midwives were by my side right up until they transferred me to Cardiff.

I will forever be grateful to the staff who looked after me that day. My baby is now home and doing well after a week's stay in Cardiff. I regularly think about all the staff who work in Carmarthen and I am eternally grateful to all of them.

Coming home was particularly difficult, as the people I needed most to love support and help us weren't around to come and comfort me in my time of need, and with everything going on. I think the hardest thing was having to get someone to come and have my other children while I was in the hospital and travelling back and forth to Cardiff. Luckily, my Sister in Law who was also pregnant had been shielding so she offered to help us by having them.

Despite all that's going on the after care has been brilliant. Even though they were having to wear all the PPE the Midwives and Health visitors have been brilliant, and I cannot thank them enough.

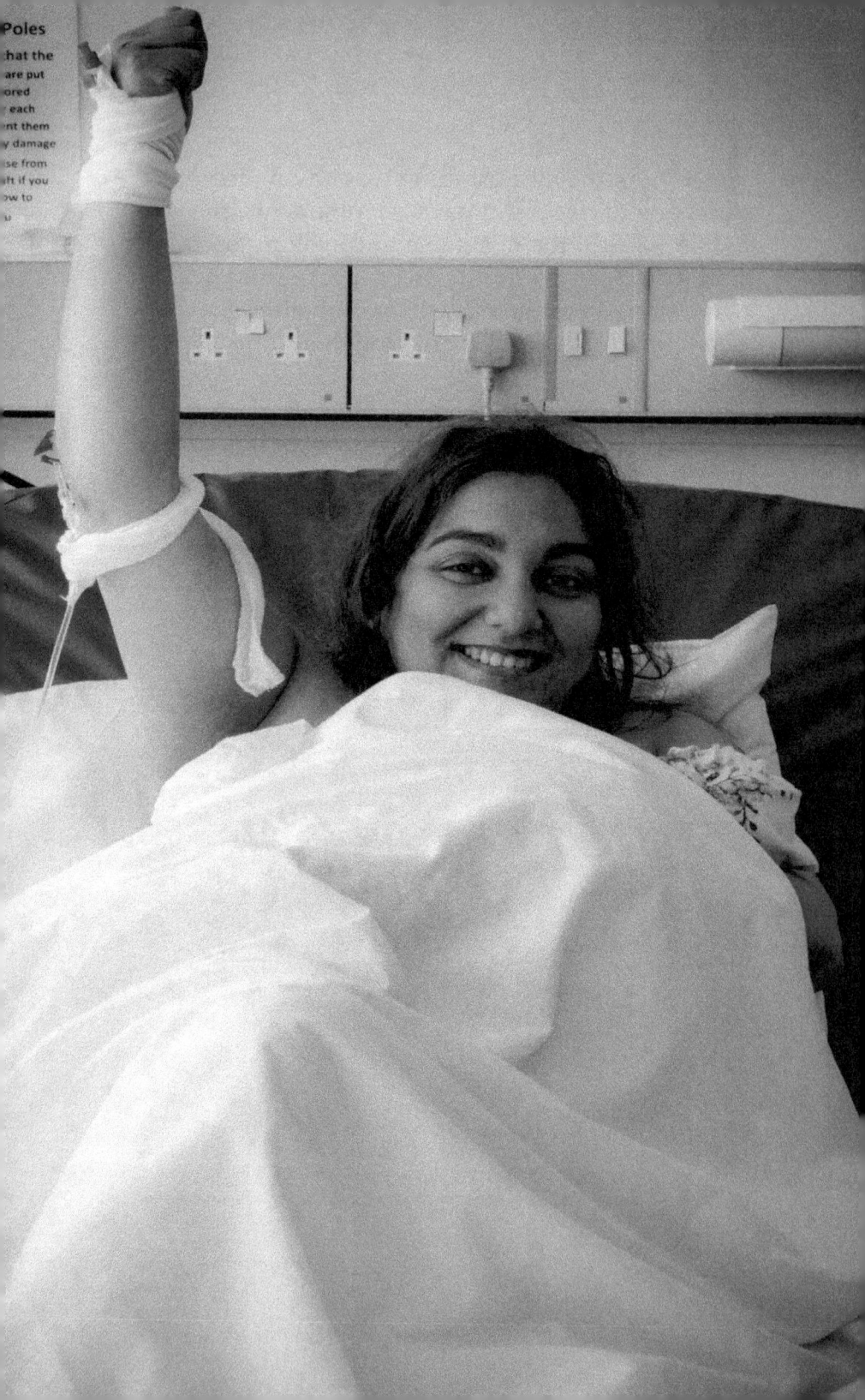

No. 25

Amanda's Story

My name is Amanda and I have the most amazing seven-year-old little boy. After a few hard years of finally completing my degree, starting my dream job, battling anxiety and trying to balance being a working mama and a professional career; we finally decided to expand our family. I stopped taking my birth control in July 2019 and had no idea what to expect as it took us a while to conceive with our first. Being a planner, I was hoping to get pregnant around December to February. However, pregnancy and conception do not go to plan. I found out early September that I was pregnant. I made my husband come home from work to tell him because I wanted him to be the first to know. He has wanted a second baby for a long long time. I wrapped three pregnancy tests (had to be sure!) in an envelope and handed it to him. I remember him looking at them and just crying.

We wanted to tell our son but we were scared just in case anything went wrong but the thought of waiting for twelve weeks to get confirmation was too much so we booked a private six week scan which worked out around end of September. I had no early symptoms apart from a migraine because I've never suffered with them, and I felt sick if I didn't eat little and often. Due to my anxiety I kept dreaming I lost the baby and there was no heartbeat so around the scan I was a wreck with worry! But the scan showed our little jellybean all healthy and happy and there was a strong heartbeat. I was so excited as we told our little boy he was going to be a big brother and he was very very excited! We told him with a letter and got him a T-shirt which said he's going to be a big brother. He was so excited to tell his teacher and friends, but he understood he needed to wait for our twelve- week scan, and he was so excited! However, when we got the letter, we were extremely disappointed to find out he was not allowed to go! The twelve-week scan was a relief as baby was doing well and we were able to announce our pregnancy around December 2019. We booked a sixteen weeks gender scan privately to find out the gender and so he could see the baby as he was not allowed in the other scans. Our little boy was convinced it was a girl and turns out he was right! We were over the moon.

January came and my pregnancy progressed and due to a change of job January flew by. However at the end of January covid cases were being spoken about and come February when we first started hearing about the coronavirus in the U.K. in no way did we expect how much it would escalate and the scale of its impact on our lives.

As the things progressed, we carried on being as normal as possible. However, in March 2020 as announcements were being made and cases were getting higher and higher, I started worrying about my safety and the safety of my baby as it was unknown how the virus affected pregnant women and the unborn baby. I was driving home from work when I heard the announcement that pregnant women were now under the 'high risk' category. I was very lucky my boss texted me to work from home immediately, so I was isolating from the 17th March 2020. My job as a social worker meant learning to work in a new way. However, it was not until I had a hospital appointment and had to attend on my own that I realised how horrible, scary and real the situation actually was.

I had to attend my 28 weeks appointment on my own and going into a hospital after lockdown made me realise how scared I was. I went in wearing a mask and using so much hand gel. I was shaking because people were coming in and out and had to be told to leave there as there was no two- metre distancing and my appointment was running late. My scan was 9:40 I was not seen until 11:50, then I saw the consultant at 12:40 and then had bloods after that. Leaving the hospital, I was a wreck shaking. This was my first time leaving the house and it was awful. Having bloods on my own was awful too as I hate needles and usually my husband holds my hand and talks me through it! Further appointments were just the same, the anxiety of going there and having my husband missing out on the scans was heart-breaking. Also, complications had to be dealt with on my own and waiting for reassurance from a Consultant on your own was not pleasant. On top of this I had a seven year to home school whilst working from home. I developed SPD towards the end of the pregnancy but there was no support available due to the pandemic, antenatal classes got cancelled and no online support offered.

I had a bleeding scare around 33/34 weeks and had to go in on my own petrified whilst my husband was scared in the car waiting for news. The experience was surreal; Midwives in masks and PPE, therefore for me it hit home then that this was going to be my birthing experience. I was also informed that my chosen hospital was no longer offering water births and my husband was not allowed in 100% until I was in 'established labour' and moved to labour ward and if admitted after birth there would be no visitors including my husband. I had to grieve about this because I was robbed of what I wanted and hoped this pregnancy would be. We knew this is our last child and the things I wanted done differently I will never have. My surprise baby shower got cancelled, my maternity photo shoot got cancelled, our newborn shoot cancelled, I was unable to have my hair and eyebrows done. I felt cheated! My mother upset because she will not be with me.

The thought of giving birth on my own was petrifying, I know I'm a strong person but I felt awful because my husband was missing out on the birth of his daughter too and he has missed out on so much, my son robbed of the first experience of meeting and visiting his sister in hospital, robbed of showing her off at school drop offs and pickups! Little simple things we had taken for granted but memories robbed from us. I accepted this new normal I had to. And I started seeing stories of mums giving birth and they were incredibly strong and brave women, inspiring really and for me one image became my inspiration a woman giving the middle finger with her baby captioned 'f**k you covid 19' and I knew then I could do it. Whilst robbed of some things people became more creative in what they did, I had a virtual baby shower from my amazing new work colleagues where during our weekly team meeting on Skype they all wore pink and coordinated for flowers and presents to be delivered to my door during the team meeting. It was really emotional and incredibly thoughtful. I was able to have an outdoor socially distanced maternity shoot to capture this pregnancy and whilst I did miss out on some things, I had different things instead.

I found out at a Midwife appointment that

baby was measuring incredibly large for my gestation and my level of fluid was raised. I needed to be scanned but was refused due to having an appointment the following week due to being deemed as not an emergency even though I begged to differ. Another appointment again on my own and baby was measuring 9lbs 1oz at 37 weeks and high fluid levels. The Consultant luckily agreed with me and arranged for an early induction the following week at 38 weeks and so the plan was induction to commence on Monday 4th May 2020 at 4pm or a caesarean-section on the Thursday if the induction process failed.

I finished work on the Friday 1st May, I had planned to have some special quality time with my son but alas it was not meant to be. Monday came and all packed and ready to go but it was awful. My parents came to see me and were terribly upset they could not even hug me. My son was upset that he couldn't visit me for God knew how long. It was surreal going in on my own and frightening. Everyone in masks, gowns it was eerily quiet too.

Despite this, I got in my shared room and despite being upset leaving our threesome behind because we were about to become four. I met the people on my ward, and it was lovely to see other adults and have company. I met the Midwife as well that delivered my son nearly eight years ago, that was lovely I did not expect that. My induction started straight forward, and I was ticking along slowly. The second pessary I lost down the toilet literally and therefore had the gel on the Wednesday as I couldn't have another pessary. With the gel there were some concerns, given that I was contracting. I consented to the gel and within an hour I was in terrible pain and the Midwife whom was in charge of my care was the Midwife from the day before so she was familiar with me and concerned at how much I was contracting and sought the advice of the Doctor. I needed a muscle relaxant injection to stop the contractions however until this kicked in and the gel wore off, I had to ride it out.

This was when I realised the reality of my situation and how awful it was, and I become incredibly emotional. I wanted my husband there with me to just hold my hand and rub my back and wipe my tears. My Midwife came in with me and talked me through if she helped me breathe, encouraged me and held my hand. She reassured me through each contraction and found me a tens machine to help with the pain and not once did she waver in her support. I was terribly grateful for her and the human contact as the contractions were intense and I was not allowed much pain relief at this point. Much to my dismay I was still only 2cms but there was nothing else they could do for me so I had to be moved onto labour ward as they could reach my waters but it had to be broken by a consultant.

Once on labour ward my husband was allowed to come in and it was a long night. The experience was great and nothing there felt out of the ordinary apart from the masks. My care was outstanding. My Midwife spoke to me, asked me my choices and respected them. She laboured with me and reassured me and my husband at every point. My labour then progressed 'naturally' as can be expected considering my waters had to be broken and she listened so well that she found out the Midwife that delivered my son was on duty the following morning and managed to get her over to delivery so that she was able to deliver our daughter as well as she felt it would make a great birth story for them both and it did. I was very grateful. My new Midwife came, and we laboured and progressed, and our baby girl was delivered all 8lbs 12ozs of her and we were so wrapped up in her and we were given time to bond with her and take her in. I was asked to stay in for a further period of monitoring. This was not what I wanted but going back to post-natal ward was lovely actually. I never thought I'd say that, but I had quality time to bond with my little girl in a quiet ward and got to know her further and rest.

I held her, got wrapped up in her and for a few hours my sole focus was her. There were no distractions of visitors just me and her and it was exactly what I needed. I was taken care of by some lovely people and we got discharged the same day. My little boy came with his Daddy in his mask to get his sister and got to meet her for the first time. This was beautiful to witness and I'm grateful that he got this at least. Our family sadly were unable to meet her and her Grandparents met her through the car window and socially distanced garden visits when the weather allowed but they were not allowed to hold her due to the risks. This was sad and I don't think I realised how upsetting this was going to be. My friends were unable to meet her as well and even though we bonded as a family and adjusted well to the lack of routine and nowhere to go was hard. Every day feels like Groundhog Day. My parents finally met her and held her for the first time when she was eight weeks old. There were lots of tears.

Postnatally I found more challenging actually due to the support being limited. I wanted to nurse her but unfortunately was unable to latch her. The first midwife that called out went through everything but later on I couldn't put her back on. I asked for further help and when the other midwife called out to see us, she was amazing and took her time and showed me a few things. My daughter fed beautifully but again I was unable to put her on myself pain free. I started pumping to express milk when it came in and fed her that. However due to lack of stimulation from her I am only able to get one full bottle feed a day 4ozs of expressed breastmilk in her. I have since reached out for support from breastfeeding experts as miraculously my daughter is still willing to latch but I cannot put her on in any way to achieve a deep latch that is pain free. Video support whilst great does not work for me. This has left me feeling like a failure as a mother as she was/is quite poorly on formula screaming crying due to colic, constipation and reflux. Some days she'd cry so much that I would sit there crying with her. Because of this I have been putting her to breast for comfort with a shallow latch and pushing through the pain to offer comfort but some days I'm too sore from blistered, bleeding nipples.

I feel this has been the worst part for me because I wanted our feeding journey to be different especially as she wanted the breast whereas my son did not. I feel robbed and cheated out of so much, but this hurt the most, because it's labelled 'easy and natural' when it's extremely difficult. I am disappointed that I will not again experience this and have had to grieve about the loss of this because this was something I longed for.

Despite it all I gave birth to the most beautiful little girl and got my 'f**k you Covid' picture and did it. Women are amazing and we really can do anything. Whilst this was not the birth plan I had in mind when we got pregnant and yes experiences were robbed and things were so far from different there was no way to predict or guess how it would could have been. There were still things to be grateful for and those are the things I'll remember. these are what I'll hold on to.

I want to Thank all the Midwives that risked their lives to make us safe and have these experiences; for being thoughtful and considerate to ensure it was memorable, especially for me. We were able to recreate the same image with the Midwife for our daughter just like our son and how lovely it will be to tell them that whilst it could have been anyone it wasn't. We were fortunate to have the same incredible person bring them both safely into the world. If anything, this strange time has allowed us to slow life down really focus and reconnect. Showing us that really all that matters is being kind, caring and compassionate. How strong we can be when we're forced to be. What really matters is love and family. Everything else fails in comparison. When you strip it all away it really is all about the simple things in life that make us happy and happiness is a choice, we need to make every day. Thank you to everyone that helped to complete our family. Covid 19 did not destroy this for us. We have our girl and now three became four.

Conclusion

It has been an absolute privilege to compile this collection of Birth Stories, they provide a valuable insight to the true experiences of the women who have lived this totally unusual event of giving birth during a global pandemic. This unique situation of the coronavirus brought a time of both worry and uncertainty for them all.

Social distancing, national lockdown and hospital visiting restrictions meant the women had to miss out on all of the normal opportunities, like having company to go for antenatal and scan appointments, having Grandparents visit for precious first cwtches, and being able to proudly show off their newborn s to their friends and family.

But, to the absolute credit of all the women who gave birth during this pandemic, the stories reveal that the unprecedented conditions were accepted not only with good grace but without objection.

Despite the unusual circumstances, and the disappointments at having to sacrifice so many of the emotional and special moments with their families, the stories also demonstrate how the women recognised the positive side of lockdown, with more valuable time for treasured family bonding, and the privacy to establish feeding.

"...we were put on lock down! I was faced with questions such as "Is my husband allowed to come to the appointments?", "Is my husband going to see our first child being born?" answers that would all soon come to light..."

"It's now the beginning of 2020, it s the first time we hear about the coronavirus on the news. I remember watching the news and thinking to myself it s so sad what these people are going through in China and Italy. I never imagined it would ever reach us here."

"The lockdown affected my mental health more than anything, knowing that all the plans I had for when baby arrived can no longer be carried out, my parents still haven t met their granddaughter, it s difficult."

"Since this coronavirus has taken over it s been quite difficult, more so for my partner, who had been very hands on during the pregnancy. So, for him not to be able to come to any more antenatal appointments was hard."

"When it came out on the news couple of months later that pregnant women are at high risk and they need to be isolated for three months. That is when reality hit me."

"I still felt safely distanced from other people and the wonderful level of individual care was not affected by the current health situation."

"After hearing about the covid-19 I noticed things started to change. I was receiving letters to go to antenatal appointments, but they were different this time I was asked to attend on my own."
"After completing the monitoring checks, we phoned my partner at home, put him on speaker phone, and completed my birth plan together. Whilst not what we had expected, it still allowed both of us to be part of the discussion and ask questions."

"From my perspective on both experiences all I can say is, that all births are epic journeys, and all mothers are warriors however they birth, and each birth was a personal Everest for me."

"The Midwives were all wearing gloves, mask and plastic aprons but their eyes and their words all conveyed reassurance, humanity and compassion."

"But there is no doubt that there is a feeling of lost time, because my maternity leave has a finite end date. There is a chance that my Baby girl will never get to experience mother and toddler groups, not see another baby, before I have to go back to work"

"There have been advantages, the lockdown has meant that we have been able to settle into a routine for us. The lack of visitors is hard in some respects,

we don't know when the Grandparents will be able to meet their Granddaughter and give her cwtches, we haven't been able to meet our newborn niece who lives in London. In others, it has been a revelation. No visitors meant no constant interruptions, and feeding has been easier to establish. No school runs meant we've been able to adapt our routine around the baby's needs, without making my 7-year-old feel like she's an inconvenience."

"Being told I could push at last was the most wonderful thing. Pushing and birthing my baby was a truly awesome, powerful experience."

"The Midwives and Health Care Assistants were marvellous, they came every time I pressed the buzzer and helped me with baby and were very good at telling me that I was doing a fantastic job and taking it all in my stride. I needed the encouragement."

"I couldn't have my mum there for support during the birth due to restrictions on only having one person. I also couldn't have the photographer present to record the birth either. Everything I had envisioned was taken away due to covid-19."

" am five days postnatal and no one except my midwife and my children have seen our son. My stepchildren have also been affected as they have yet to meet him and we have no idea how long it will be before they get to meet their little brother and have their first cuddle, None of my friends or family have met or cuddled him."

"So everything changed, three months ago I would have said you were mad if you told me I was going to give birth at home in my pool without any pain relief and just with my partner and a Midwife. However, the experience in itself was beautiful, calm and serene. Being at home I had all my home comforts, and two hours after giving birth I was cuddled up in my own bed looking at my miracle, The support from the Midwife couldn't of been better and she kept me relaxed throughout the entire experience."

"I totally understood but I couldn't help feeling upset, scared and worried. I was devastated when I found out only one birthing partner, I would have loved to have had my mum there for the birth. I had Tears rolling down my face knowing that I couldn't have my mum there holding my hand for the birth."

"Not able to have visitors into the hospital. Most importantly not seeing my fiancé while we stayed in hospital for a couple of days after the birth. Everything felt so unnatural emotions were high."

"I had two lovely Midwives waiting there for me. I felt relief that I was there, and I felt safe. It was quiet, not another patient around, I walked into the ward and my lovely Midwife made me feel very comfortable. From that very moment, I felt okay."

"It all felt so natural like nothing was going on

in this world. Yes, they were wearing gowns, gloves and they even had masks on, but I respected that for all of our safety. The days went by, and everything was so professional and relaxed. I didn't feel anxious at all, I knew we were in the right care."

"Even though, it is only normal to feel upset and lonely not having my family around me when I needed them the most. I didn't feel like I was on my own, I was in the best of hands and I cannot thank them enough."

"Then on the last few appointments there was tape placed across seats to ensure people were sitting the correct distance apart, Midwives and Nurses wearing face masks and disposable aprons."

"His birth hasn't really been celebrated as I've not seen anyone to celebrate, My baby shower was also cancelled, so all the presents my friends and family got for him will have to wait till after lockdown in order to receive them."

"The one positive to covid-19, is that we had time to bond as a family and it s been nice to not have to worry about people visiting and being able to just relax and enjoy our first few days."

I hope you have enjoyed reading these Birth Stories. I wish to extend my gratitude to all the women and their families who so generously shared their stories.

"Thank-you"

As this book goes to print, national lockdown restrictions are steadily easing, however there is a lot of discussion about the potential for a second wave of the virus in the months to come. The use of face-mask coverings is becoming more widely used and already compulsory in some areas of the UK. Some hospital visiting restrictions remain in place and quarantine regulations have been introduced for some foreign travel.

It feels like the Covid -19 story may be far from over...

www.ingramcontent.com/pod-product-compliance
Lightning Source LLC
Chambersburg PA
CBHW071125240526
45465CB00024B/1083